TRY
DRY

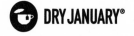 DRY JANUARY®

THE OFFICIAL GUIDE TO
A MONTH OFF BOOZE

TRY
DRY

WRITTEN BY LAUREN BOOKER
FOREWORD BY LEE MACK

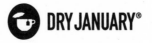 DRY JANUARY®

SQUARE PEG

1 3 5 7 9 10 8 6 4 2

Square Peg, an imprint of Vintage,
20 Vauxhall Bridge Road,
London SW1V 2SA

Square Peg is part of the Penguin Random House group of companies
whose addresses can be found at global.penguinrandomhouse.com

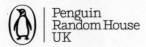 Penguin
Random House
UK

First published by Square Peg in 2018

penguin.co.uk/vintage

A CIP catalogue record for this book is available from the British Library

ISBN 9781910931998

Typeset by Anna Green at Siulen Design

Printed and bound by Clays Ltd, Elcograf S.p.A.

Penguin Random House is committed to a sustainable future for our business,
our readers and our planet. This book is made from Forest Stewardship Council®
certified paper.

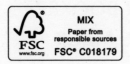

CONTENTS

FOREWORD

I grew up in a pub in the 1970s on a council estate in Blackburn. The regulars were serious drinkers. Not serious in a 'they don't smile' sense, as they used to smile a lot. But the kind of smile that only heavy drinkers do. The one where it looks like someone has just told them something hilarious but there's actually nobody sat next to them.

I can tell you now the regulars of the Centurion on the Roman Road estate would have viewed Dry January with a great deal of suspicion. 'A month off the booze? Why?' Although if they were more honest with themselves they would have said, 'How?' Because to these regulars, having a month off the booze would have been tricky to say the least. They would have struggled with Dry Thursday. In fact, Dry Breakfast would have been a challenge for some.

I have sort of done Dry January myself. I say 'sort of' because I stopped drinking alcohol on 3 January 2017. I wanted to stop on the 1st and do a proper Dry January. But the problem I had was that I knew I was going to the PDC World Darts Championship Final on 2 January (Michael van Gerwen beat Gary Anderson 7–3 if you're interested. No? Oh, just me then). And starting the first couple of days of not drinking by going to the darts is a bit like starting your diet by visiting the Jammy Dodger factory. So I had one final blow-out and decided to stop for a short while. I had no intention of stopping completely, I just wanted to have the rest of January off the booze. But because I'd slightly cheated and not done 1 or 2 January, I made myself do an extra couple of days in February so I could say to myself that I'd done a month. And then I thought, 'Oh well, I've started February,

I may as well see it out.' And before I knew it February had become March, and March had become April, and April had become May and . . . well, I'll let you take it from here, you know the order of the months, right? And here I am, a couple of years later, and I've still not had any booze.

And I guess the question you're thinking is, 'Yeah, but how much were you drinking?' I say that because whenever I tell people how long it's been since I had a drink I always get The Look. The Look is when people want to say, 'Were you a normal drinker who decided to just get a bit healthy, or were you regularly waking up in a skip with your trousers missing?' But they can't ask that, because it's awkward, so they always play safe and nervously say, 'Oh! What made you do that?' which covers both. And I sometimes think they are hoping to get the trouserless skip anecdote, because that way they can think, 'Ah well, I'm not like you, I'm a normal drinker so I don't need to do it.'

For what it's worth I think I would have been classed as the normal type. You know, a glass of wine in the evening in front of the telly. Well, maybe two. And I guess they were fairly big ones. And occasionally I might finish the bottle off. And there was the odd blow-out where I'd get a bit legless, like at Christmas. And New Year. Oh yeah, and birthdays. And get-togethers with old mates. And on holiday. And stag dos. And Friday nights. And Saturday nights. Like I say, normal.

For me the appeal of drinking was the altered state of mind, whether it was to feel more relaxed, or feel more social, or feel more carefree. But one day I just had this sudden urge to have a different altered state of mind for a change and see what it was like to not drink at all, for a proper amount of time, not just a couple of days. I suppose I was just curious. What does it actually feel like to be a complete non-drinker? Even if it's just for a month?

So, how did it feel? Well, sort of tricky at first. The first few days were easy. It's like the first few days of getting fit or dieting. You're full of enthusiasm for this new-found, life-changing attitude. But by day three or four you start missing it a bit. You have a stressy day, you open the fridge, and staring back is a cold bottle of Blue Nun (OK, it wasn't Blue Nun, it was actually a decent bottle of Sauvignon blanc. But I'm the kind of person who's always had this terrible fear of becoming showbizzy and middle-class, perhaps because I've got one eye on being offered the Greggs advert. You know the type, those awful people who can't even do a foreword for a book without mentioning that they grew up on a council estate in the first sentence). So it was a struggle at first. And I did wonder if I could be bothered carrying on. Then I had a bit of an enlightening moment.

On about day four of not drinking I was in a pub with a mate. This was my first day in a pub since the darts night several days earlier, so I knew it was going to be a struggle not to have a drink. I decided to compromise with myself and have a non-alcoholic drink to start, and then see how I felt afterwards. If I really fancied a pint after, I'd have one.

So I bought a lemonade, and he ordered a pint of lager. We'd both had a stressy day writing jokes (you're probably sat there with your proper stressy job, thinking, 'Writing jokes? Stressy? Get a grip, mate.' Well, all I can say is, you're wrong, it's stressy). He took his pint, drank some, did that exhale of relaxation you do when you have that first sip, looked instantly calm, and said, 'That's better.' And after the initial wave of jealousy that only a man drinking Sprite looking at a man drinking beer can feel, I suddenly thought, 'Hang on, that can't be the alcohol making him instantly relaxed, it surely takes longer than that for it to get in the bloodstream (at least 30 minutes apparently). There must be something else going on here.' The fact that it was the first time he'd sat down all day, and was drinking an ice-cold drink, and was no longer working, and maybe *that's* why he felt instantly relaxed didn't occur to him. But it hadn't occurred to me either for the previous 30 years.

That's what made me carry on not drinking. Not the health reasons, not the idea of living longer, and not because my local shop has stopped the three-for-two deal (although that was a motivation). But because I realised the whole thing is just a bit of a con.

If you're reading this, you're probably thinking about having a crack at a dry month. Well, good for you. What have you got to lose? It's only four weeks and three days. Or 744 hours. Or 44,640 minutes. Or 2,678,400 seconds . . . actually, this isn't helping, is it?

And if you're the kind of drinker who thinks, 'Yeah, but I'm alright, I don't drink that much. I'm certainly not addicted' (i.e. pretty much everybody), then you're the perfect person to Try Dry. Because it will be a doddle. Right?

Lee Mack

ABOUT THE AUTHOR

Lauren Booker is an alcohol consultant for Alcohol Change UK, the charity behind Dry January. Having worked in the field for over fifteen years, Lauren has an encyclopaedic knowledge of all things alcohol and, more importantly, has a lot of experience helping people to change their relationship with it – whether that means moderating, cutting booze out for a month or going alcohol-free longer term. With her invaluable expertise, Lauren is the very best person to lead *anybody* through their booze-free journey.

INTRODUCTION

Millions of us barely let a week go by without toasting, taking a tipple or just downright glugging our way through the days, so it can be hard to imagine a) why you'd want to go dry for a month and b) how on earth you could actually do it.

Yet every year around four million people in the UK try Dry January, taking a month off alcohol to reset their relationship with booze and get a whole host of other benefits. Foregoing their nightly tipple, even just for a few weeks, helps this lucky four million to lose weight, sleep better, look better, reduce anxiety, gain more energy and, of course, save money.

'But *how* could *I* do it? A whole month off booze?' I hear you cry, through a glass of Pinot and a bag of nuts, teary and confused by my plan to RUIN your social life. Well, that's where this book comes in.

I'm going to be your guide and companion, or Dry Guru, if you will, as we navigate this booze-free journey. Why me? Because I've trodden this path before you and emerged sober and happy at the other end. I've also led many, many other people down said path over the last few years in my role as resident alcohol counsellor and consultant for Alcohol Change UK, the charity behind Dry January. Basically, you're in safe hands.

These pages will cover every stage of your dry journey, from 'coming out' to friends and family, to sex and relationships, setbacks, cravings, going out and staying in. I hope you'll find personal stories to inspire you and a wealth of resources that can help to smooth the path through your own personal dry challenge.

I've set this out as a month-long journey because a month is a good amount of time to reassess your relationship with alcohol. It's also an easy amount of time to remember, so hopefully your friends and family will be able to keep track of how long they'll have to put up with your glowing skin and new positive outlook. It's long enough for you to experience lots of normal 'life' stuff like pay days, minor crises, weekends and birthdays of friends, and short enough for you to see the end in sight.

Having this one-month goal is like having a destination; you know where you're aiming for, and that will help keep you going. Plus you'll be able to set landmarks along the way – 'my first weekend dry', or 'halfway there'.

Another reason for taking on a month-long challenge is because **it takes just three weeks to break a habit**. Some are ingrained, but with just a little bit of focus, we have the power to change our habits for ever.

This challenge is all about you. To start with, you get to choose which month you want to take off. January can be a good time; it comes right after traditionally boozy December (so you're probably sick of the stuff anyway), you're setting New Year's resolutions, and a whole lot of other people are going dry with you for Dry January. But it doesn't have to be January – you can choose any month of the year, and this book will help you to pick your month to maximise the benefits you'll feel.

You don't even have to commit to a month. If you want to try a couple of weeks to begin with, feel free to use this book to help get you started. But as I said above, it's a good idea to set a goal to keep you motivated.

You don't need to read *Try Dry* from beginning to end all in one go. I recommend you start by reading chapters 1 and 2, but after that just go wherever your fancy takes you. You can go back to sections that you find particularly helpful and redo the quizzes to see how your answers change over time. This is **your** book. You can use it in any way that you find helpful. It's up to **you**. Write your name on the inside front cover if you want. There, feels just a bit naughty writing in a book, doesn't it?

Words from the wise

Throughout the book there will be stories from other people who have done a month alcohol-free, pulled out in bold. These are bona-fide Real-Life People who have shared their stories with the Alcohol Change UK team, though a few of them asked us to change their names. Some of them will crop up throughout the book, so you can get to know them. They've got tips, tricks and anecdotes to keep you going.

SO WHY GO DRY?

Trying Dry can be really transformative for anybody at any stage of their life – whether you're a busy student, a young professional, a knackered parent, or a finally free retiree. There are lots of reasons why so many of us take this challenge and everybody will have their own story. What would yours be?

'I was having a knee operation and wanted to cut down drinking before it.'

'I wanted to lose a bit of weight.'

'Just to do it, stick to it for the month and feel better.'

'This gives me some control. I have suffered with depression in the past and I know alcohol can relate to that.'

'To change habits and make sure when I did go back to drinking, I would drink significantly less often, and less overall.'

Here are some of the most common motivations for people taking a dry month (or more). Stop for a moment and have a think about your year ahead and whether any of these apply to you – you'll want to have a few up your sleeve for page 21. Having a motivation like one of these in mind is a good idea. When the going gets tough, the motivated get going.

YOU'RE BUILDING UP TO A BIG EVENT

Wedding of the year? Tropical holiday? Whatever the special occasion, you want to look your best and that means bright-eyed, clear-skinned and full of beans. We've got just the thing. Just one month without alcohol and you're likely to be able to tick off all of the above. Plus you'll save some cash to put towards the big event.

YOU DON'T LIKE YOUR RELATIONSHIP WITH ALCOHOL

What might have once been a love affair with the sparkling, witty person you become after a drink or two has turned into leaning on booze just to get you through the evening. If it's become more habit than fun, a month off is a good way to reset. The skills and tricks you learn along the way – how to say no when someone offers you a drink, how to go out and have fun booze-free, how great it feels to wake up on Sunday morning without a hangover – are what makes a dry month so worthwhile, even long after the month is over.

YOU WANT MORE ENERGY

Who doesn't want more energy? It's surprising how daily drinking can sap your 'get up and go' and leave you lacklustre and constantly fuzzy in the head. With no alcohol, you'll get higher-quality sleep, and it will be less interrupted as you make fewer visits to the loo. If you want to feel years younger in just four weeks, yup, this should do it.

YOU WANT TO LOOK BETTER

Since heroin chic went out of fashion, there's no mileage in the sunken-eyed, grey-pallor, hangover-from-hell look. Fresh-faced is in. If you were considering microdermabrasion, a facelift or wearing a paper bag for the foreseeable future – good news! Cutting out alcohol can make a bigger difference than you imagine.

YOU'RE PREGNANT OR TRYING TO BECOME PREGNANT

This is a big one, isn't it? If this is you, you've got a fabulous motivator.

There are plenty of useful 'not tonight' excuses in Chapter 3 to help you keep this secret. When you do share the happy news, trust me, no one will be offering you a drop of the hard stuff.

YOUR PARTNER IS PREGNANT OR TRYING TO BECOME PREGNANT

Just because you're not actually carrying the future prime minister/star striker/world-famous cancer-curing doctor doesn't mean you don't have a role to play at this stage. Your partner will find it soooo much easier to avoid the booze if you're not stocking up the fridge with tinnies every weekend.

If you're taking the challenge to support someone for another reason, it's a great way to show you care.

SOMEONE ELSE HAS SUGGESTED YOU CUT BACK

This is an eye-opener, isn't it? You're thinking you're the life and soul and your mates are thinking, to quote Captain Jack Sparrow, 'Hide the rum!'

Maybe they've been subtle, *à la*: 'Ooh, it might be nice to not drink for a while – what do you think?' Or maybe it's more: 'You're a lush. Get a grip.' Either way, take the hint. If you find yourself defending your drinking habits – what does that tell you? So take it personally, but in a good way. A dry month lets you evaluate your drinking from a sober perspective.

YOU'RE RAISING MONEY FOR A CHARITY

Maybe you've lost someone to alcohol and want to raise funds for a charity like Alcohol Change UK, the organisation behind Dry January. Or maybe you'd like to raise money for another charity. If this is you, try not to look too smug but yes, you should be proud of yourself.

Or how about pledging? If the idea of asking friends and family for cash fills you with horror, why not pledge some of your savings instead? After all, the cash you would have spent on drinking this month is free dosh, right?

YOU HAVE HEALTH CONCERNS OR YOUR GP HAS SUGGESTED A CHANGE

Uh-oh, wake-up call. This is a great opportunity to make a change. Check out Chapter 5 to see all the ways your body and brain will thank you for giving them some time off alcohol.

YOU'RE TRAINING FOR A SPORTING EVENT

Go you! Whether it's your first Park Run or the London Marathon, I absolutely promise that this will make your training easier. Alcohol is a muscle relaxant so the more you drink, the harder you have to train to get those pecs pumped and those glutes, er, gluting.

However, as wonderful as the benefits of a booze-free month can be, I do understand it's not the answer for everybody . . .

REASONS NOT TO TAKE A MONTH OFF ALCOHOL

It's all well and good me telling you about all the great things coming your way when you go for a month without a drink (I did mention saving money, weight loss, bright eyes, fresh skin, clear head and better sleep, didn't I?), but are there any reasons not to try a month off?

Yes, of course there are. Here are a few situations where it's not a good idea to take on the challenge.

I WANT TO GO COLD TURKEY

Check out the warning on page 10. If you are currently drinking very heavily, it can be dangerous to stop drinking suddenly. For most people this won't be the case, but if you're concerned please do check. Done? OK, read on.

IT WILL SOLVE ALL MY PROBLEMS

No it won't.

Yes, we rave about the benefits of a month off, but it's not a magic bullet. It can set you up for other positive changes but don't think that this is all you have to do to deal with the problems in your life.

However, if you use the now-free drinking/hangover recovery time to work on relationships, reflect on your choices and seek solutions, it can certainly set you up for a better year. How do I know? Been there.

If you've been sticking your head in the sand – or rather the glass – and using booze to distract you from your problems, quitting drinking is going to bring those problems into sharp focus. You might benefit from starting to work on the other issues first and then use a dry month to consolidate the changes that you make.

MY FRIENDS/FAMILY DON'T THINK I CAN DO IT SO I WANT TO PROVE THEM WRONG

Why don't they think you can do it? Are you one of those dynamic people who is always starting projects that fizzle out after a few days? Do they think you'll lose interest in it? Are they planning to sabotage your month? You'll find that taking on the Try Dry challenge is much, much easier when you've got support from friends and family (and even easier if they're doing it too).

It's not always a bad idea to Try Dry if you want to prove your family members wrong – but you do need to **be sure that you're doing it on your terms**, because it's a great thing to do, but not just because you've been teased into it.

If you're sure you are doing this for you but your family and friends are still doubting, why not get them to put their money where their mouth is and sponsor you? That'll shut them up!

MY PARTNER/PARENT/CHILD/OTHER LOVED ONE (DELETE AS APPLICABLE) IS MAKING ME DO IT

If you're going to commit your energy and focus to this challenge, you need to be doing it for the right reasons. **It has to be because you want to** and are prepared to put in the time. If you feel bullied or coerced, don't do it. You won't enjoy it, it'll be harder to stick to, and ultimately it won't improve your wellbeing if you feel resentful about not having a drink.

It might be useful to think about why your loved one is so keen for you to stop drinking for a month. What's in it for them? Are they worried about you? Talk to them about their concerns and your reasons for not wanting to take up the challenge. Having a frank, open discussion about how you both feel can clear the air. Try to see things from each other's point of view.

If your loved one is concerned that you're drinking too much and this is their way of asking you to slow down – do they have a point? Complete the quiz in Chapter 2. If you answer the questions honestly, and your score is over 15, then it might be wise to think about ways that you could change your drinking to reduce your health risks (more on that in Chapter 5). But if you're still not up for a month off, take a look at the resources section on page 210. There are lots of other ways that you can cut down your drinking.

If you do decide to Try Dry remember – you need to do it for **you**.

I THINK I SHOULD DO IT BUT I DON'T REALLY WANT TO

Why do you think you should? If you're worried that your drinking is getting out of control, even just a few days without a drink can seem really daunting. If you go into this challenge with the belief that, even if you don't want to do it, a month off will make your concerns go away, you're not alone. But you *are* fooling yourself.

Get any health concerns checked out with a medic. Get any relationship concerns checked out with your loved ones. Read the book. Work your way through all the activities in Chapter 1 and if, hand on heart, you still feel more *should* than *want to*, stick the book back on the shelf and come back to it later.

Do come back though; trying a dry month because you really want to can be a very powerful thing.

WARNING: For some people it can be dangerous to stop drinking suddenly . . .

. . . but only if you are heavily dependent on alcohol, which could be the case if you drink heavily and regularly. If you think that this could be you, or if you have any other health concerns about either your levels of drinking or giving up, please see your GP before you go any further. I mean it. Get it checked out.

If you don't want to talk to your GP you can contact your local alcohol support service for advice. You can find a local services directory on Alcohol Change UK's website alcoholchange.org.uk.

You can also complete the AUDIT quiz (a questionnaire developed by the World Health Organization to work out how risky your drinking is) in Chapter 2 to see whether your drinking is at potentially dependent levels. Even if you don't score that highly, if you struggle to go a couple of days without a drink or you have any symptoms when you stop – DO NOT DO THIS CHALLENGE. Go to see a health professional and get some help to make the changes you want to make.

ARE YOU IN THE ZONE?

Now the reasons *not* to Try Dry are out of the way, let's check where you're at.

Here's a little quiz to see how highly a dry month ranks on your to-do list right now. I understand you might still be wavering . . .

Circle the number of the statement that best represents how important it is to you at the moment to conquer this challenge.

1. I don't actually want to do this at all, I'm just reading my mate's book while they're in the loo.

2. It's not at all important, I'd rather climb a mountain or tame badgers as a challenge.

3. I'm curious, but only theoretically curious, not actually-do-it curious.

4. I'm not really bothered, but I could give it a go as there are no badgers or mountains in the vicinity.

5. It's a good idea, but I'm not committed.

6. I keep thinking that this is the way to go, I'm just not sure when.

7. I want to do this, I can see the benefits, but what if I find it too hard?

8. I really want to do this; I'm willing to try.

9. It's become much more important to me over time. I'm ready to commit.

10. Can't wait! Sign me up, I'm ready.

Let's take a look at your score.

If you circled 1 or 2, then this probably isn't the right time for you to try this. Did you buy this book for yourself or did someone give it to you? Maybe someone around you thinks that you'd benefit from making a change in the way that you drink, but you don't necessarily agree. Well, that's OK, a dry spell isn't for everyone.

This might not be the right time but don't rule it out in the future. Put the book back on the shelf and pick it up again in a month's time. Circle a number again – if your answer has changed, read on.

If you circled 3–5, you may have reasons for thinking that a month off alcohol would be a good idea but you can't see yourself doing it at the moment. It would be great if you could just wave a magic wand and experience the benefits without having to actually stop drinking for a month, right? This is where most of us start.

Don't put the book down just yet. Read through the next chapter. It will give you ideas for making changes and help you to decide whether a month off alcohol is right for you. It will also highlight some of the benefits that haven't even crossed your mind yet. Even if you decide that now is not the time, don't throw the book away. You might want to give it a dry in future (or at least come back for the great puns).

If you circled 6–8, you're hurtling towards the decision to give a dry month a try but you're not quite there yet. What would raise your response to a 9 or a 10? What needs to be in place for this to be important enough for you to make the commitment? Spend a few moments thinking about this.

Now read to the end of Chapter 1 and then come back to this page. Has your number gone up?

If you circled 9 or 10, you've already made the decision, you just have to get your plan in place and get on with it. When a goal is this important to you, you have a very high likelihood of achieving it.

Read some of this book every day. Pick a chapter that you think will help, read one of the reflections from fellow dry travellers, or complete one of the quizzes.

The secret to maintaining your momentum through the month is to keep your focus on your goal. Choose the bits of the book that you find most useful and turn to them whenever you need a boost. You've got this.

Right. Are you ready to get started?

1. MENTAL PREPARATION

Introducing . . . Me, Myself and I

Me: I wonder what it's like, not having a drink for a month.

Myself: Dunno. Never tried. It's not like we drink a lot. Not during the week, anyway.

I: Yes we do. We had a drink last night.

Me: That's right. We weren't going to, but there was that open bottle and it's a shame to waste it, so we finished it.

Myself: Yes, but that's not every night.

I: It's more often than not, these days.

Me: Eek.

Myself: It's not just us, you know – everyone does it.

I: No they don't.

Me: Don't they?

I: Nope. According to the Office for National Statistics, less than 10 per cent of UK adults drink on five or more days a week.

Me: Should we be worried?

Myself: Yeah, alkie, bet we couldn't stop if we wanted to.

I: Sorry to interject but we probably can and we might even enjoy it.

Myself: No we won't.

Me: We might. We can do without the weekly hangover.

Myself: Nothing that a couple of paracetemol and a morning in bed can't take care of.

Me: And we'd save a bit of money.

Myself: One time, just *one* time we lost our wallet on a night out and you never shut up about it.

I: Then there was that incident with our new phone.

Myself: That wasn't because we were drunk, that was because we were dancing on a roundabout in the rain, after midnight, recreating the iconic tableau from *Flashdance*.

I: The prosecution rests, M'lud.

Me: Good point. Where do we sign up?

CONCERNS AND CONFIDENCE

If you're ready and raring to go – brilliant. But if you're not feeling so positive, that's normal. Another important factor in taking a month off booze – and in any life decision – is confidence. Here are some of the most common worries that our community of Try Dryers have expressed:

WHAT IF I CAN'T MANAGE THE WHOLE MONTH?

Drinking is a solid part of your routine, your kids are named Chardonnay and Shiraz – and that's just the boys – so you don't think you can last the month . . . Well, so what? How about if you manage a week? How about if you go for a drier-than-the-last-one month? It's *your* challenge, you can do whatever you like with it. Just don't use this as an excuse for not starting in the first place.

Obviously, aiming for the full month is a good place to start. But if a day comes along where your boss has a meltdown, your team loses at home to Fulham and you have a blip, well, it's not the end of the world. In fact, it'll help you prepare for things that might cause slip-ups in the future. If you do have a drink, you'll go back into the month better armed to face any other obstacles. For more on this, check out Chapter 7 on setbacks.

I'M WORRIED THAT I'LL JUST DRINK MORE WHEN THE MONTH IS OVER

One of the funny things about taking a month off is that it doesn't make you want to drink more 'to make up for it'. In fact, as your body gets used to no alcohol, it's not keen on you starting again. So the first time you do have a drink, take it easy – it can hit you pretty hard.

It's up to you what you do, of course, but most people find that having experienced the highs of an alcohol-free month, they don't want to go straight back to their old drinking habits. You'll also have learned a tonne of new skills to help you have a happier relationship with alcohol in future – skills like how to say no to a drink you don't fancy and how to have fun at any event without booze (though I reckon you secretly have this skill down already).

In fact, research has found that 72 per cent of people who attempt a Dry January have a lower AUDIT score six months after their dry month than before they did it.[*]

I'VE GOT A SPECIAL EVENT COMING UP (BIRTHDAY/WEDDING/HOLIDAY) – WHAT DO I DO?

Go! Enjoy! Have a fabulous time! And do it all without the risk of overdoing the booze and forgetting the unforgettable occasion,

---

[*] De Visser, R., 2016, 'Voluntary temporary abstinence from alcohol during "Dry January" and subsequent alcohol use', *Health Psychology*, vol. 35, no. 3, 281–9.

without the nausea, without the hangover, without wondering what you said to whom after a few too many.

Plan the event out in advance (see Chapter 10 for some great ideas) and start thinking about how great the experience could be without a drink rather than how it might not live up to your expectations.

I KNOW WHAT MY WEAKNESSES ARE; WHAT IF I CAN'T BEAT A CRAVING?

Cravings are normal. They're to be expected. And they're easy to tackle if you know what to look for and what to do when they hit. You can find some really useful tips on how to tackle cravings in Chapter 6.

Now, let's do some confidence building.

➜ Dust off that trumpet; think of something you've achieved that you're proud of and write it here. It can be anything at all.

➜ What makes you so proud of this? How did you do it? Write down the skills that you used here.

→ How did you overcome the obstacles? Jot down some of the ways you rose to the challenge.

→ Think: how can you use the skills you talk about above to take on the Try Dry challenge?

Stu

'You get the sense from the some people that they'd love to try it, but they don't think they could. What's the worst that can happen? You can fail on day one, sure. You can try again in a couple of months, there's no barrier to stop you from trying it as many times as you want.

—

Feeling more confident?

Me, Myself and I on motivation

Me: We might lose some weight and get back into our jeans.

Myself: Not likely, not with our on-going sugar addiction.

I: Well, maybe a little weight.

Me: We could stick the cash we save in a jar and treat ourself to something flashy.

Myself: Yeah, or raid it for a box of chocolate fingers every couple of days.

I: Great idea, Me, we could put it towards a holiday.

Myself: No way we're getting in a swimsuit.

Me: Well, we might sleep better.

Myself: Not a chance with our stress levels!

I: We'd feel less stressed after a couple of weeks without booze.

Myself: Still won't sleep though. Betcha.

Me: Know what I'm most looking forward to about our month off?

I: Myself not being so bloody grumpy all the time?

Myself: Good point.

Janeska

'I became self-conscious of my drinking when I had to take my daughters to kids' parties, often on a Saturday morning. I'd find that more and more I was telling the other mums I was chatting to that I was hungover from our Friday date night the night before.'

—

MOTIVATION

I know, I know, we already talked about the things that might be motivating you to go dry, but now it's time to get specific. Trust me – getting specific, personal, positive motivations worked out will be a huge help to you throughout the month.

That word – positive – is so important. If you think this is going to be a slow, painful, uphill slog, where you feel deprived and miserable – stop the negativity. It won't help you. Stop it; stop it now. **You can transform your relationship with alcohol in a positive way.** You have the **power** to not only take a month off booze, but to enjoy the ride too.

Make a list of all the reasons you're doing this. All of them. Psychologists say that writing our goals down makes us more likely to commit – so get scribbling.

Try to think about what you want to gain, not what you want to ditch. 'I want to lose weight, sleep better and have more time at the weekend,' works better than 'I hate my beer belly, my sleep pattern is shit and I want to avoid hangovers.' If you're thinking, 'I can't afford to keep drinking,' you could reframe this as: 'I'm saving for something important.' We're much more committed to our goals when we're working towards something than when we're trying to move away from something. Except when running away from a tiger (or any other large, fast-moving carnivore).

Identify the positive outcomes that will come from your motivation for an extra motivational boost!

→ Insert your motivations here:

Motivation	Positive Outcome
I want to sleep better and look more fresh-faced	I will feel more confident when I turn up to Ben's wedding looking fabulous
I want to learn to be in control of the amount I drink	I'll have fewer hangovers and get my Sunday mornings back. Hello, brunch!

Now, rank these in order of importance. Why? Because if you understand why you're doing this (and I mean on a deeper level, not just 'I'm broke 'til payday so it's give up booze or biscuits') it'll be easier for you to stick to.

Take a look at your list and focus on how you'll feel when you achieve all these wonderful things. Yes, you'll probably lose a bit of weight and save a bit of cash but how will you *feel* when you succeed? Write that down too.

Now stick your top three reasons and how you want to feel where you will see it every day. You could make it the screen-saver on your phone, or stick it to your fridge, or have it tattooed on your arm – just make sure it's going to be visible every day for the next month!

FUTURE YOU

So. You've gone through the whole of Chapter 1 and you're still here. You've decided to take the plunge and give up alcohol for a month. After the month where do you hope you'll be? What message do you want to send to the you who's completed 28 (or more) alcohol-free days?

I've written to future me a few times about goals I've had. I get Mr B to post these notes to me at the end of the challenge. I've usually forgotten about them by then so it's a nice surprise. Am I the only one who still gets excited about any post that doesn't come in a brown envelope? Thought not.

Even if you don't want to post it, fill in the postcard on the next page. Tell yourself how proud you are. Let yourself know how you're hoping to feel. Don't peek until the challenge is over. You'll get to see how far you've come, and have someone who believes in you (you) telling you how well you've done!

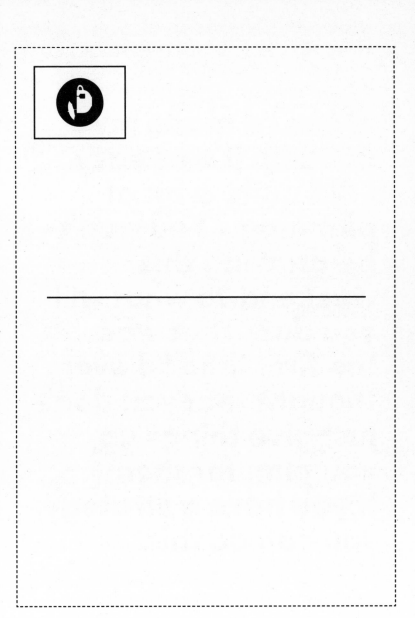

Cadence

'Once I'd made my mind up it was easy. I did quite a bit of planning. "You won't be drinking this weekend so what will you do?" That was the first time I'd ever thought that you don't just give things up, you plan for them. If you have a strategy, you can do this.'
—

2. GETTING STARTED

COUNTDOWN TO QUIT DAY

Here we are then. You're feeling motivated and ready to go. What happens now?

Good question.

First of all, a bit of preparation is in order. You know the old adage – fail to prepare and you prepare to fail. Well, this is never truer than when it comes to making lifestyle changes.

HOW MUCH ARE YOU DRINKING AT THE MOMENT?

It's a good idea to see what your drinking patterns are like at the moment. Maybe you think you're drinking too much or too often or maybe you're just not sure – so let's find out.

In the UK, alcohol is measured in units. A unit is simply 8mg of pure alcohol. If you look on the back of any alcohol label, you'll see the number of units in the bottle/can. You can often find the number of units in a single serving too.

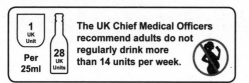

1 UK Unit

Per 25ml

28 UK Units

The UK Chief Medical Officers recommend adults do not regularly drink more than 14 units per week.

If you want to work out the units in your drink from its strength, there's a calculation you can use. Just multiply the volume of your drink in millilitres by the strength of the alcohol in per cent (that's usually represented by the letters ABV or 'alcohol by volume') and divide the whole answer by 1,000.

(ml x %ABV) ÷ 1,000 = units

Here's an example:

One pint is 568ml, and let's say we're looking at a lager at 5 per cent ABV so:

(568ml x 5) ÷ 1,000 = 2.84 units

Simple, huh?

If the idea of dusting off your abacus doesn't appeal, there are lots of less medieval ways of working out units. How about downloading a drinks tracker app to do the job for you? There are quite a few free ones out there, including the Dry January app. This handy little thing allows you to track not only your alcohol consumption but your spending on booze and calories consumed too. It will also check in with you to see whether you've stayed dry. Take a look in the resources section at the back of the book for more app options.

HOW MUCH BOOZE IS TOO MUCH BOOZE?

The government has issued guidelines for low-risk drinking. Ideally we should all stick to a maximum of 14 units a week, most of the time. That's about a bottle and a half of wine, five pints of standard lager or seven double spirits. Of course, it's better to spread that over the week rather than drinking it all in one go. That's also a maximum by the way, not a target to hit. You don't have to drink anything at all! It's a good idea to have two or three days off a week.

→ Over the page is a quiz that looks at your current drinking and some of the ways it might be affecting you. It's called AUDIT (Alcohol Use Disorders Identification Test) and it was developed by the World Health Organization. It's used worldwide to give people an idea of how their drinking measures up risk-wise. It's a really simple and effective way to find out whether the amount of alcohol you drink could be putting your health at risk.

Answer all the questions then check out your score on the next page. No cheating – after all, no one is going to see this but you. If your score is higher than you thought it would be, don't blame the AUDIT. This little quiz has been proven time and time again to give an accurate picture of the level of health risk your drinking brings with it. Take it on the chin and then Try Dry.

Questions	Scoring system					Your score
	0	**1**	**2**	**3**	**4**	
How often do you have a drink containing alcohol?	Never	Monthly or less	2–4 times per month	2–3 times per week	4+ times per week	
How many units do you drink on a typical day when you are drinking?	1–2	3–4	5–6	7–9	10+	
How often have you had 6 or more units if female, or 8 or more if male, on a single occasion in the last year?	Never	Less than monthly	Monthly	Weekly	Daily or almost daily	
How often during the last year have you found that you were not able to stop drinking once you had started?	Never	Less than monthly	Monthly	Weekly	Daily or almost daily	
How often during the last year have you failed to do what was normally expected from you because of your drinking?	Never	Less than monthly	Monthly	Weekly	Daily or almost daily	
How often during the last year have you needed an alcoholic drink in the morning to get yourself going after a heavy drinking session?	Never	Less than monthly	Monthly	Weekly	Daily or almost daily	

Questions contd.	Scoring system					Your score
	0	**1**	**2**	**3**	**4**	
How often during the last year have you felt guilt or remorse after drinking?	Never	Less than monthly	Monthly	Weekly	Daily or almost daily	
How often during the last year have you been unable to remember what happened the night before because you had been drinking?	Never	Less than monthly	Monthly	Weekly	Daily or almost daily	
Have you or somebody else been injured as a result of your drinking?	No		Yes, but not in the last year		Yes, during the last year	
Has a relative or friend, doctor or other health worker been concerned about your drinking or suggested that you cut down?	No		Yes, but not in the last year		Yes, during the last year	
					Total	

Your score

If you scored **0–7** this is the low-risk category. This means that you're unlikely to experience any harm to your health from your drinking if you continue to drink at this level. Still, going dry for a month won't hurt and you're sure to notice some benefits.

A score of **8–15** means that there is some risk from your drinking. Everyone is different, of course, but I'll bet most of your points were scored on the first three questions. That's because the drinking comes first and the problems come later. Although on the whole booze doesn't interfere that much with your life, you may be ready to make some changes and an alcohol-free month will kick start your new pattern of drinking.

If you scored **16–19** you're already aware that drinking has a downside. It's likely that others have commented on your drinking or it's starting to creep up to a level that you're not comfortable with. Well, that's why we're here! Taking a month off will help you to 'reset' your drinking to a lower level or pave the way for longer-term changes. It will give you a chance to step back and look at what you might want to change in the future and, most importantly, you can do that without the interference of booze in your brain.

A score of **20+** can mean that you're becoming dependent on alcohol. This is a lot more common than you might think. You can certainly turn things around but you'll benefit from some outside support. Have a word with your GP or contact your local alcohol support service (visit Alcohol Change UK's website for a directory of your local services) to see what your options are before you continue with this challenge. Once you've had the go-ahead from a medic, come back and join us. Taking a break from alcohol will give you an opportunity to reflect on how you want to proceed. Lots of people in this position take their dry journey beyond the first 30 days, others 'reset' their drinking to a different level.

Whatever your score on the AUDIT quiz above, if you've got any doubts about your suitability for trying a dry month, for example if you're a daily drinker, please consult a professional. And no, I don't mean a bartender. There are times when it's not appropriate, or safe, to stop drinking.

The Four Ls

You're definitely drinking too much if you've got problems with one or more of the four Ls:

LOVE – is your drinking having a negative impact on your relationships? This might be arguing with your partner, missing time with your kids, your mates not inviting you out because you're embarrassing when you've had a few, for example.

LIVELIHOOD – are you late for work or taking duvet days to recover from hangovers? Not getting assignments in on time? Passed over for promotion because you're not as sharp as you used to be? Starting to notice that you're the only one who heads to the pub at lunchtime?

LIVER – . . . But not just your liver. How's your health in general? If you've got high blood pressure or cholesterol, are overweight, experience anxiety or depression or just generally feel bleurgh a lot of the time, drinking is not helping.

LAW – if you drink and drive and kid yourself that it's just a couple of drinks and you'll be fine, or you've actually got a conviction for drink driving; if you've been arrested for being drunk and disorderly or get kicked out of venues because of your drunken behaviour – yep, I'm talking to you.

WORK OUT WHAT KIND OF DRINKER YOU ARE

Different drinking patterns will need different strategies if you're going to get through 28+ days without giving in to the temptation of 'your usual'. Pick the description below that most closely resembles your drinking style. If you're not sure, show this page to a good friend – what kind of drinker would *they* say you are?

The Weekender

It's Friday night and the weekend has landed. You don't make plans for Saturday or Sunday because you know you'll be out partying 'til the wee hours and recovering well into the afternoon, when you'll be ready to hit the town again.

Not drinking during the week won't be a problem for you. You can happily go Monday to Thursday (or possibly Wednesday) without a drink, but you work hard and reward yourself with a lively social life at the weekend.

If this is you: There are two things that might trip you up on your dry journey:

1.   You don't want to miss out on any fun and you're going to feel deprived if you don't get your weekly fix of drinking your fill.

2.   You think everyone has expectations that involve you knocking back the booze and being the life and soul of the party.

What can you do to prepare? Take a look at the Try Dry reasons you listed in Chapter 1. Do they still hold true? If so, treat your four alcohol-free weekends as an experiment. You're there to observe what the world in general and going out in particular is like without an alcohol haze.

It can be daunting to think of having a good time without a drink. After all, can you even have fun sober? The answer, of course, is yes – but nevertheless, be prepared to temper your social life, just for this month. Going out sober can take a little bit of getting used to – though once you do I bet you'll have a better time than ever. Chapter 10 will help you get the party started minus booze.

If you're worried that your friends won't stick around if you're not part of the drinking gang, take a look at Chapter 3 for some tips on how to get them on side.

The Daily Tippler

You mostly drink at home or at your local – somewhere you feel comfortable and relaxed. You have a drink most nights, your usual drink, your usual number of drinks and your loved ones know your routine. You don't necessarily know why you drink – you just do.

You're rarely drunk and you won't feel the desire to go out and get hammered very often, but it's become a daily habit and it makes you feel a little bit out of sorts if you break your cycle.

If this is you: Your stumbling block is breaking out of that routine and finding something else to fill the space. You can't imagine how you're going to fill a whole month of evenings if you can't have a drink.

What can you do to prepare? Well, the good news is that it can take just three weeks to break a habit. However, a good plan is of the essence, because if you find yourself at a loose end you're likely to head for the comfort of the bottle/can/glass and your favourite armchair/barstool.

Is there an evening class you've always wanted to take? A dog you can walk? Could you rediscover your love of underwater basket weaving? Just shifting a few little things can help to break you out of that comfort zone. Try sitting in a different chair or a different room. Hit the bar at a different time, or a different bar, or no bar at all. Coffee, anyone?

If you feel yourself thinking about a drink – have one, just not an alcoholic one. As you plan, spend some time checking out local pubs and bars' alcohol-free drinks or browse your supermarket for something refreshing. Some people like to choose an alcohol substitute, while others prefer avoiding all thoughts of alcohol. Try a few different things so that when D-Day hits, you've already got a new favourite drink.

As a daily drinker you're more likely to experience cravings than the weekender so it's a good idea to take note of the pointers in Chapter 6.

The Both Ends of the Candle-er

Every day is a party day. You seem to be able to go out any (or every) night of the week and still get up bright and early the next day.

You're an excellent host; your parties are legendary. If you're drinking, you like everyone around you to be drinking. More booze = more fun. Something's got to give, though.

If this is you: You may feel it's time to slow down and take things easy for a while, but what if it's just boring? You might struggle with the idea of spending time sober, possibly with your own company.

What can you do to prepare? If you use alcohol to socialise, it can be hard to figure out how to spend your time and who to spend it with when you're not drinking. Do you think your friends will struggle with the idea of you going alcohol-free as much as you will?

Who do you know that doesn't drink, or doesn't drink much? Come on, you must know someone. Why not spend some time with them before you start your challenge? Find out what they do to have fun. Plan a couple of evenings with them.

If you do intend to go out during your challenge, you may find the temptation to drink is overwhelming. Hanging with drinking friends can be tedious if you're not on the same level. Tell your drinking buddies beforehand that you're not imbibing. Take the car so you can't drink. Choose a venue that has a range of mocktails/alcohol-free beers/food. That way you can still feel as though you're joining in.

Be prepared though; you may have to make significant changes in order to stay dry. Keep your goal in mind; remember why you want to do this.

The quizzes in Chapter 4 (especially 'Fill the Gap') will be particularly useful.

The Unwinder

You drink to unwind, to forget the troubles of the day and because, goddammit, you deserve it. A drink in the evening signals the end of the working day/week and you use alcohol to relax. During particularly stressful periods you have a drink (or two) to help you sleep.

If this is you: When things are going well, you won't think about booze much, but what will you do if there's a crisis?

What can you do to prepare? You need to explore other ways of relaxing before you head into your dry month. Experiment with warm baths, playing your favourite tunes, yoga, PlayStation, gardening – the options are infinite. Take a look at the activities in chapters 4 and 9.

Think about the things that make you feel stressed – is it situations? People? Deadlines? Try this before you Try Dry: write the following questions down (or note them on your phone). Whenever you feel stressed or upset, go through these one by one.

What is making me feel stressed?

What can I do about the situation?

Who might be able to help?

How can I take care of myself right now?

At the end of the week, take a look at your list and think of something you could have done in each stressful situation or what you actually did that worked – unless it was a large glass of red! These are your stress-busting alternatives to booze.

It may seem as though alcohol is a quick bridge from 'worry' to 'no worry' but it's built on rickety foundations. And there's a troll living under it. Other relaxing resources will help much more reliably!

The Emotional Drinker

You drink when you're sad, bored, tired or lonely. If you're nervous in social situations, a drink will make you more out-going. If you've got an unplanned evening ahead of you, you'll find something interesting to do once you've had a drink. Maybe you're getting over an emotional break up, bereavement or other loss and alcohol helps you to forget the negative emotions for a while.

Jess

'Temporarily stopping is a good way to feel your emotions and to recognise the why behind your drinking. It surprised me that when things got a little bit stressful or after certain conversations I couldn't wait to have a glass of wine and I thought, "Well, maybe there is that emotional component and I should check out for a while."'

If this is you: You're in a rut and drinking helps you to stay there. You're going to have to climb out and tackle the touchy-feely stuff that you've been avoiding by hiding behind a glass – and that can be hard.

What can you do to prepare? Practise the mindfulness activities in Chapter 4. This will start to get you thinking about your triggers for drinking. Once you've identified exactly how you feel when you reach for the glass, you can start to work on strategies for responding differently to that emotion.

Complete the checklist of things that you can do instead of drinking in Chapter 4 ('Fill the Gap'). Chapters 9 and 10 also have some great ideas for keeping busy throughout the month.

Rest assured, a month without alcohol should help with both mood and sleep. If you're really struggling to make changes and your mood is usually low, it might be worth a visit to your GP.

YOUR PRE-TRY DRY TO-DO LIST

Those are the basics. Now let's get started on some logistical planning in the form of a to-do list. Why not tick them off as you go along?

1. CHECK YOUR CALENDAR

When are you going to start your challenge?

As I said before, January can be a really good time, especially if this is your first dry month, as so many people will be going dry right along with you. Pubs, bars and restaurants are geared up with alcohol-free options. Besides that, you might still be nursing a hangover from the festive season.

But it really doesn't have to be January; any month will have its own challenges and opportunities. Take some time to think about when you're going to start the clock. If you've got a really huge event coming up that you know you're going to want to enjoy with a drink (think landmark birthday, collecting your OBE, anniversary of the opening of Krispy Kreme's 1,000th concession), don't start your challenge three days before. Yes, you can enjoy these events without a drink, but why pile the pressure on for your first ever month off?

Get out your diary – do you have a four-week period coming up that is relatively light on big events? Don't wait for a completely blank month. The idea is not to become a hermit for four weeks, only venturing out when the pubs are shut, under a cover of darkness. Christenings, weddings (other people's), nights out with the girls/lads, leaving parties – all these can be enjoyable without booze. In fact, the challenge is to embrace such events, have a fabulous time, and watch your mates go green with envy at how fresh and sparkly-eyed you look the next day. Just be realistic and choose a month with some events, but not too huge and not too many.

It will help to start your challenge on the first day of the month (if you're going for a full 30/31 day month) OR on a Monday (for 28 days).

Psychologically, either of these will give you a boost. It also makes it easier for you to check how much of the challenge you've completed. Imagine: after day one there are just three more Mondays to go, or by the 10th of the month you're a third of the way through your challenge. This is a useful tool for keeping your motivation up.

Some things to think about when picking your Try Dry month:

- Is this a relatively stress-free period?

- Have I got time and inclination to start my planning now?

- Will I have time during the month to read the book and complete some activities?

- Is this a good time for those around me?

- Will this fit in with my existing commitments?

- Whatever happened to David Hasselhoff? Is he still around?

Try to leave at least a week between reading this and the first day of your challenge. There's tons of stuff for you to do in the meantime. You want to be well-equipped for your alcohol-free month.

→ Once you've decided on your date, write it down on your Try Dry challenge plan on page 204.

Your Try Dry challenge plan

Flip on through to the back of this book, to page 204. This is where you can record details of your month for a two-page roadmap and motivational boost. Some of the activities in the next couple of chapters will help you get the info you need to fill it in. Also there's a handy list of 'Thoughts for the Day' that you can work your way through.

Now tick off every day as you count down to day one, and complete some more of the activities in this chapter and Chapter 3.

2. GET APPY

Anna

'I absolutely love the Dry January app. I have never been able to abstain from alcohol for this long before.'

Why not download the free Dry January app? Whenever you're planning to Try Dry, in January or any other month, the app will give you lots of support along the way. You can track your units, money and calories saved by not drinking and get articles on all things alcohol year-round. It's available on the App Store or Google Play.

Whether you want to count units or calories or use your new-found free time racking up steps on a pedometer, there's sure to be an app that will help you. There are some suggestions in the resources section on page 210.

3. COUNT YOUR SAVINGS

You'll be surprised at how much you can save just by not buying alcohol for a month. Thinking about this ahead of time can really help with your motivation. Why not put aside the money you save to treat yourself to something at the end of the month to celebrate your achievement?

And I do mean treat yourself. You are absolutely not allowed to spend your hard-won cash on new windscreen wipers for the car, toys for the kids, getting the washing machine fixed, etc. This is more like lottery winnings (OK, maybe I'm exaggerating a bit, but you get the point). This is money that you would have otherwise drunk and have nothing to show for other than a few blurry pictures on your phone and a month of hangovers. Enjoy your new wealth.

→ Let's work out how much you'll be saving. Fill in the drink table below. Don't forget to work out your drinks on a night out – you probably pay more per drink than if you're drinking at home.

Fill in your total savings on your Try Dry challenge plan on page 204.

What I drink	Where I drink this (e.g. home, pub, club, mate's house)	How much does one drink cost?	How many times I have this drink each week	My weekly saving (column 3 x column 4)
Medium glass (175ml) wine				
Large glass wine (250ml)				
Bottle wine (750ml)				
Can of cider, lager or other beer				
Bottle of lager, cider or other beer				
Pint of lager, cider or other beer				
Single spirit (e.g. vodka, gin, rum)				
Double spirit (e.g. vodka, gin, rum)				
¼ bottle of spirits				
½ bottle of spirits				
Cocktail				
Fortified wines (port or sherry)				
Other				
	TOTAL SAVING PER WEEK:			
	TOTAL SAVING PER MONTH (total per week x 4):			

In reality, you may save a lot more than this if you're not drinking. Taxi fares, late-night kebabs, overgenerous tipping – it all adds up. Not to mention getting a round in, which can often be more than you bargained for.

Of course, you're likely to be spending some of this money on other things – alcohol-free alternatives, activities in the evening and at weekends which involve more than just a bottle. But I bet you'll still spend less, and you're likely to have a lot more to show for it.

Cadence

'When I finished I had my hair done and it turned out beautifully. I had saved £14 (the cost of two bottles of prosecco) every week. I bought a pair of expensive shoes and I remember wearing them and feeling so proud of myself.'

—

4. CHUCK THE BOOZE

That's right – ditch it. Empty your house of alcohol. Completely. The easiest way to avoid temptation is, well, not have it there in the first place.

Having alcohol lying around makes it much more likely that you'll decide to have a drink. It's easy enough when you're in the planning phase to think, 'No, I won't, I can do this whether there's a six-pack and a nice bottle in the fridge or not.' Well, maybe you can, maybe you can't, but why put yourself through the test if you don't have to? It's for that very reason that I don't keep cake in the house. If it's there, I'll eat it. No cake has ever gone stale under my roof.

Not willing to pour your Moët & Chandon down the sink? No problem. Just find a drinks-sitter for the month. Someone who will store the contents of your drinks cabinet and won't give in to any late-night pleading for just one quick can of ice-cold cider. Make sure it's someone you trust to a) not drink it themselves; b) be supportive of your goal; c) give it back at the end of the month.

If you can't ship the booze out to a friend, how about stashing it somewhere tricky to get to? I'm thinking in the loft, or the shed at the bottom of the garden, or the very back of that nearly jam-packed cupboard?

While we're on the topic, it can be cathartic to get rid of the booze you're never, ever going to drink. Hands up if there's an untouched bottle of ouzo or banana liqueur lurking at the back of a cupboard. We've all got one. It's been there since Aunt Ethel's trip to Corfu in 1994. Trust me, if you haven't found an occasion to drink it by now, you never will. Empty it out and recycle the bottle. There: you're saving the planet, too.

5. GET A GROUP

Going it alone can be tough so why not go dry with a buddy? There's lots of research to suggest that completing a challenge is easier and more enjoyable if you've got company. Going dry is the new black, so there's bound to be a kindred spirit in your circle who's up for giving it a go. Seriously, just drop into conversation that you're going to give dry a try and you'll soon find someone who's been thinking the same. Then check out Chapter 3 for some ideas for going dry as a group.

Your buddy doesn't even have to be physically there. There are lots of great sober/semi-sober online communities of people sharing their experiences and providing a lifeline for if you have a bit of a wobble. Check out the online communities in the resource section.

6. TELL YOUR TRIBE

Who are you going to tell about your challenge? There may be some in your social circle who won't take you seriously. They may tease or tempt or downright sabotage your dry month. Others will be supportive from the outset. Trying Dry can teach you lots about your friends and family! So be prepared. Check out Chapter 3 for some great tips on how to handle telling different people.

ARE YOU READY, WILLING AND ABLE TO START YOUR DRY CHALLENGE?

You've completed all the activities above and in Chapter 1. Now it's time to find out – are you ready, willing and able to tackle your dry month? You're going to need to be all three of these to keep your momentum up for the length of your challenge.

Stu

'If you drink quite a lot you tend to not experience what a hangover is anymore because it just becomes part of the morning. And two to three weeks in, I was getting straight out of bed, being more productive – that is a nice side effect. All of a sudden you think, "Wow, these hangovers made me lose two to three hours of my day."'

—

Are you READY, WILLING and ABLE to start your Dry Challenge?

You'll need to be all three to keep up your momentum for the length of your challenge.

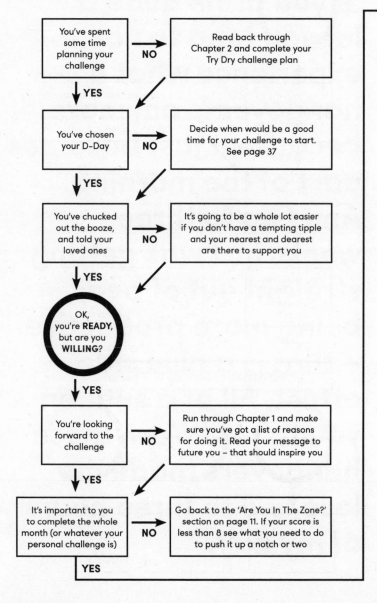

You've spent some time planning your challenge → **NO** → Read back through Chapter 2 and complete your Try Dry challenge plan

YES

You've chosen your D-Day → **NO** → Decide when would be a good time for your challenge to start. See page 37

YES

You've chucked out the booze, and told your loved ones → **NO** → It's going to be a whole lot easier if you don't have a tempting tipple and your nearest and dearest are there to support you

YES

OK, you're **READY**, but are you **WILLING**?

YES

You're looking forward to the challenge → **NO** → Run through Chapter 1 and make sure you've got a list of reasons for doing it. Read your message to future you – that should inspire you

YES

It's important to you to complete the whole month (or whatever your personal challenge is) → **NO** → Go back to the 'Are You In The Zone?' section on page 11. If your score is less than 8 see what you need to do to push it up a notch or two

YES

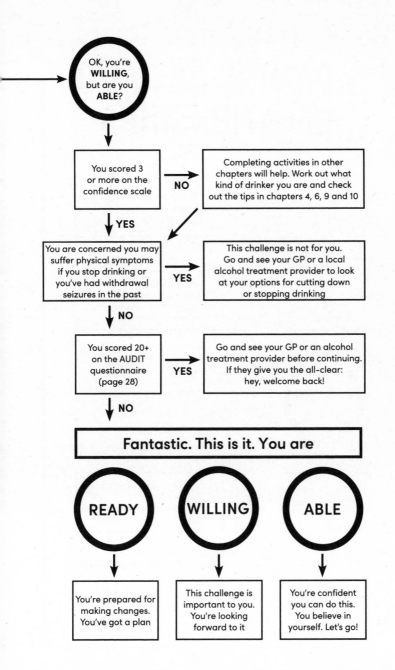

OK, you're **WILLING**, but are you **ABLE**?

You scored 3 or more on the confidence scale

NO → Completing activities in other chapters will help. Work out what kind of drinker you are and check out the tips in chapters 4, 6, 9 and 10

YES ↓

You are concerned you may suffer physical symptoms if you stop drinking or you've had withdrawal seizures in the past

YES → This challenge is not for you. Go and see your GP or a local alcohol treatment provider to look at your options for cutting down or stopping drinking

NO ↓

You scored 20+ on the AUDIT questionnaire (page 28)

YES → Go and see your GP or an alcohol treatment provider before continuing. If they give you the all-clear: hey, welcome back!

NO ↓

Fantastic. This is it. You are

READY ↓ You're prepared for making changes. You've got a plan

WILLING ↓ This challenge is important to you. You're looking forward to it

ABLE ↓ You're confident you can do this. You believe in yourself. Let's go!

3. COMING OUT AND RELATIONSHIPS

You're about to start your dry month. You've done your prep. You're ready and raring to go.

The night before you're planning to go off the sauce, you go for some drinks with friends/work/your ten-pin bowling club. Over the course of the evening you're offered at least five drinks – and maybe you accept because, after all, you haven't started your dry month yet. But it gets you thinking – how, during your dry month, would you tell all these people about your challenge? Do you want to tell them? If you don't, what *should* you say?

As much as your dry journey is about *you*, I'm afraid you're bound to encounter at least a few other humans during your month and they will have a bearing on how you experience it. Some of them will make things a lot easier and more fun, some will be curious and others may do their best to get you back to your old ways.

In this chapter, we'll look at how your relationships can affect your month off. We'll cover everything from 'coming out', to drink-refusal skills, to dealing with naysayers.

If you have a partner, they're likely to have the biggest impact on your month of anyone you know (except you), and dating alcohol-free can take a bit of getting used to – so we've got a whole other chapter dedicated to love and sex. Flip on through to Chapter 8 when you're ready.

WHO ARE YOU GOING DRY FOR?

For yourself, right? You want to feel better, sleep more soundly, save money . . .

But, as I said above, it's not always *just* about you. You might be going alcohol-free to support your partner, or to raise money for a charity or to reclaim your weekend so you can spend more time with the kids. Even if these aren't your main reasons, I bet you can think of a few people who will benefit from you and your improved mood – and thinking about them might help strengthen your resolve.

→ Jot down who you think your challenge will have a positive effect on and what that might be.

My dry beneficiaries	What's in it for them

Deb

'I was kind of excited to tell my son. Throughout the month he would say, "How's that Dry January going?" which was really great. I also told my colleague who I travel with and she started doing it too, which I didn't expect. It was like an informal, "I'm going to join you" and that ended up being really impactful for me to keep going. In fact, she's still doing it.'

Sam

'I think it's important to tell people in the weeks leading up to it. You will always have some friends who'll say, "Come on, you can have one." If you haven't mentally prepared your friends that you're doing it they're more likely to try and push booze on you in a social way.'

COMING OUT

Maybe you'll be shouting about Trying Dry from the rooftops (or at least on social media), or maybe you'll only want to tell your closest friends and family. Choosing who to tell (and when and how) ahead of time can boost your chances of success.

That said, telling people that you're going dry – especially if you drank quite a bit before – can be daunting. Welcome to your 'coming out' phase.

SO, WHO ARE YOU GOING TO TELL?

You've already made a list of the people who are likely to benefit from your alcohol-free month. Now it's time to think about who you're going to tell about your challenge. This may or may not include people on your list.

→ Use this space to think about who you're going to tell and why it's important that they know about and understand your decision.

Who I'm going to tell	Why it's important that they know

HOW WILL YOU TELL PEOPLE?

You've probably clocked by now that there are quite a few people you might want to tell. But how to do it? Obviously some people will need you to talk this through with them in more detail than others: your partner, close friends (especially the ones you often drink with) and maybe your kids. A good place to start, though, is by developing an elevator pitch.

THE ELEVATOR PITCH

The principle behind the elevator pitch is that you imagine answering a question about your Try Dry challenge – what you're doing, why you're doing it – in the time it takes an elevator (er, lift) to travel between floors. Your pitch should work for pretty much anyone: your friends from work, the guy you usually see at the pub, your nosy neighbour who's wondering why your recycling bin is suddenly so empty.

Why is this useful? Having a couple of sentences planned is great for three reasons:

1. Fake it 'til you make it. Just saying the words can help you to focus on your goal.

2. Others are less likely to question your challenge if you sound convincing.

3. Having a set response means you're not going to stumble over your words or start justifying your reasons.

The trick is to figure out how to explain your dry journey as succinctly as possible. You'll need to include exactly what your challenge is and why you're doing it. There are four steps to the perfect elevator pitch:

1. **Tell them what you're doing** – one month alcohol-free – but also why. People will want to know what's in it for you, so sell the benefits.

2. **Keep your language positive** – this is a challenge, not a punishment.

3. **Keep it brief** – this is not a justification or an explanation, just your way of letting people know. You can always lengthen it for certain people if necessary.

4. **Practise your pitch out loud**. No, really. You need to feel comfortable saying the words and you need to run through it a few times to remember what it is you're going to say. Feel free to write it on your hand if it will help.

Take some time to get the wording of your pitch right, then note it down on your Try Dry challenge plan when you're happy with it.

Here are some elevator pitches that have worked for other people:

- 'I'm enjoying a month off alcohol because it will help me get in shape for the summer.'

- 'I'm not drinking at present and it's really helping me focus on other things.'

- 'I won't be drinking alcohol between now and next month. I'm experimenting to see if it helps my training.'

- 'I'm raising money for my favourite charity by going dry for a month.'

- 'I'm having a break from drinking – it's helping me to save for my wedding/new mortgage/upcoming trip to Butlins.'

FIND YOUR SUPPORTERS

Who will be the biggest help during your challenge? Maybe you've got a teetotal cousin who can point you to bars with the best alcohol-free range, or a sibling who will keep you on track and not let you off with giving in halfway through. Perhaps you've got a mate who'll bet a substantial amount of money that you don't see the month out, making you more determined than ever.

Even better – has anyone you know done Dry January or another sober challenge? An estimated four million Brits took part in Dry January in 2018 so you're bound to know someone who's dipped their toe in sober waters. You can ask them for tips on how to enjoy the month, and pick their brains for new drink ideas, or pitfalls to look out for. Plus they're someone to chat to if the going gets tough.

→ Whoever you think your supporters are going to be, make a record below and note down how they might be able to help.

My supporters are:	I can ask them to help me by:

Make sure you've told these people about your challenge. Add this list of supporters to your Try Dry challenge plan and go back to it if you need a boost during the month.

Mark

'I went to this party and people were saying, "You can have this night off, go on," and some of my other friends (who knew about the challenge) were saying, "No, no, he's doing this for a good cause." They can insulate you a bit from temptation.'

DRY TEAM: ASSEMBLE!

Now get your dry tribe together. These are the people who may want to join you in taking a month off. Have any of your family/friends mentioned that this is something they'd like to do? If you invite them to give it a go, it might be just the motivation they need to start their own dry journey.

Even if none of your friends have expressed an interest yet, the people on your list of 'people to tell' or supporters might want to join you when you fill them in; keep this in mind.

There are plenty of reasons, both practical and psychological, why going dry with a buddy boosts your chances of success.

1. You've got a ready-made support system if your resolve starts to fail.

2. You don't want to let them down, and that can keep you strong.

3. You've got a great reason to carry on if you're supporting someone else.

4. There's someone else not drinking alongside you when you're out and about.

5. You can share tips and advice along the way.

6. You can pledge your savings to a good cause together and raise more money.

7. You've got someone to talk to who knows what you're experiencing (and is still happy to discuss the challenge when everyone else has glazed over).

8. There may be a little frisson of competition between you to keep you interested.

9. It'll strengthen the bond between you.

→ 10. Sharing is caring.

Write down the names of anyone joining you on your journey here.

Once you've decided who you'll go dry with, have a chat about how you're going to support each other, how long for and what the extent of that support will be. You might all commit to one dry night out together each week for example, or set up a WhatsApp group.

None of your friends fancy it? Don't worry! Your dry buddies can be virtual as well as physically close. There are fantastic, supportive, motivational online support groups out there. Take a look in the resource section for some great sober communities that you could join, including the Dry January Community Group on Facebook.

WHAT IF I DON'T WANT TO TELL SOMEONE – OR ANYONE – THAT I'M DRY?

If you're going dry for a month, you have absolutely NOTHING to be embarrassed about, and no one should make you feel like you have. You're doing something to be pretty proud of: taking on a challenge that will do you, your body and maybe people around you some good. If you want to, shout it from the rooftops!

That said, you might decide that telling some people isn't worth the hassle. That's OK too. If there are people around you who are struggling with their own relationship with booze, or friends and family who may not be over the moon about your choice, then you might want to keep it to yourself. If you want to just dip your toes into dry and see how it feels before making a big dry splash and letting everyone know, give it a week and see how you feel then. Don't forget the Dry January app and Facebook group can give you virtual support in the meantime.

Not telling *anyone* is possibly not the best idea. Having some support through the month can make a massive difference. Even if your friends and family aren't super supportive, just having them know about your dry month can be helpful so they don't keep offering you drinks (though knowing might not always stop them). If you do decide to Try Dry without *anyone* knowing, it's doable but it might take a bit of subterfuge.

I find that as long as you've got something in your hand that looks as though it might have alcohol in it, people don't feel the need to keep offering you drinks. In pubs I drink tonic with ice and a slice and at house parties I get the biggest wine glass I can find and fill it with sparkling grape juice. I've even had a well-meaning party-goer try to take my car keys from me after watching me guzzle three glasses of 'wine'.

→ There are some more ready-made 'get out of bar free' cards below. Tick your top five and try to remember them – that gives you one per week and a spare.

Excuse	✔
Offer to drive	
Tell everyone you've had enough already and you need to switch to soft for a while	
Take control of the bottle – if you're doing the pouring no one will notice that you're not topping yours up	
Suggest everyone buy their own rather than getting rounds in	
Ask for tonic with ice and a slice. This works for cola, too	
Order mocktails – they look just like cocktails (go to Chapter 9 for some great recipes)	
Order alcohol-free beer. It looks and tastes the part – no one will be any the wiser, and if you like a beer this could be a nice treat!	
Tell everyone that you're saving yourself for a mega session at the gym	
Find a new favourite alcohol-free drink and rave about it to your friends – for example, how delicious is ginger beer?	
State that you're really thirsty so you're just going for water for now	
Tell everyone that caffeine is your new drug of choice and order a latte instead	
Say 'I'm pregnant!' For roughly half the population this might be trickier, but you could just keep a straight face and give it a go . . .	

DRINK-REFUSAL SKILLS

Despite not having drunk in, ooh, too long to remember, my friends and family still can't seem to get their heads round the fact that I don't drink. Not even at Christmas, not even on my birthday, not even if England won the World Cup. On penalties. This means that my refusal skills still get a regular work out.

In other words, no matter how many people you tell, or how well they see you're doing, at some point you're likely to be offered a drink. Now, you've got some excuses already for when you don't fancy telling someone you're alcohol-free. But how can refusing a drink actually play out?

When offered a drink, I usually request, 'Just a soft drink, please.' The response I'm most likely to receive is: 'Sure, there you go.' Easy.

But I do understand that not having an alcoholic drink when it's flowing freely can be a conversation-starter, so sometimes I'll get: 'Go on, have a proper drink, you're not driving/pregnant/boring, are you?' The easiest response is: 'No thanks, honestly, I'm fine.' I don't offer further information. I call that my response number one. Most often, it works.

At this point you can, of course, use your elevator pitch. This is its moment! This is why you went through the process of feeling like a twit, practising it out loud in the shower. So that's response number two.

If you don't fancy getting into it, however, you've got a few options.

Response number three: 'I've got one somewhere, actually. Now where did I leave it?' and wander off looking for your drink . . .

Response number four: 'No really, no more, thanks. I'm switching to water.'

This implies that you've already had a few, even though you know it's a few lemonades. It can be a risky strategy as they might offer you another drink later in the evening, but I use this tactic when I have no intention of discussing my drinking habits.

→ Refusing drinks is like building a muscle; the more you practise saying 'no', the easier it becomes. Use the table below to think about who might offer you a drink during your dry month and how you'll respond in return.

Who might offer me a drink/where	What I'm going to say to them
e.g. my boss/leaving party for colleague	'Just a tonic, please, I've got a lot to do in the morning and I want to be super sharp.'

I have several theories about why, despite my refusing every drink that's been offered to me for the last four years, my friends continue to offer said drinks. Here are a few:

1. **Old habits die hard.** OK, so I was the cocktail queen of 1988. What can I say, it was the eighties. However, I'm now a

middle-aged mum with a mortgage and I no longer carry my passport, toothbrush and spare knickers in my handbag in case of an opportunity that's too good to turn down or a need to get out of town in a hurry. The thing is, once you're famous for your ability to drink half the pub under the table, it's hard to shake that rep.

2. **It makes them uncomfortable.** They enjoy drinking, I don't. It's not a problem for me, I like being with my friends, whether they're drinking or not. But I suspect they're secretly worried that I'm judging them. I'm not. I'm having a good time, just without the booze. I've had mates come up to me at parties and ask how many units they've drunk. Hello?! Do I look like the love child of Carol Vorderman and Sherlock Holmes? I've got better things to do than investigate and then calculate other people's drinks.

3. **They want to tempt me off the wagon.** I had a landmark birthday recently and was given champagne, tequila and a beautiful case of wine with my name on the label. All lovely, none of which I'll drink. I try to look on the bright side – that's my Christmas presents sorted.

4. **They don't believe that I don't drink.** Somehow they assume that I only drink alone or when taken by surprise. At my birthday party, several glasses of fizz were pressed into my hands by well-meaning mates, all of which I passed on to other mates in other rooms. No harm done.

The headline here is, don't be offended if (when) people who you've told about your Try Dry challenge offer you a drink. Politely refuse, remind them of your dry month if necessary, and carry on doing what you were doing.

SABOTEURS, NAYSAYERS AND OTHER PROPHETS OF DOOM

You've made your plan, ticked off your lists, cancelled your subscription to *Real Ale Monthly* and you're ready to go when, with just a few words, someone unsupportive completely deflates you. These people will be in the minority – but that doesn't mean they're not a huge pain.

Use this section to shore up your defences against those who would tempt you, scare you, ridicule you or just plain overwhelm you with their apathy. There are a few key types, and each requires a different response.

It will be tricky if your partner falls into any of these categories. We've got advice for this in Chapter 8.

The Shamer

This 'friend' laughs out loud when they hear about your challenge and starts to list all the other things you've started and not finished, including reminding you that you wanted to be an astronaut when you were six, even though you don't like heights or small spaces. They tease you endlessly and make it abundantly clear that, in their eyes, you have absolutely zero chance of going the distance. Then they delight in telling others, so that they can laugh at you too.

What to do: Well, if this doesn't spur you on, nothing will. Stick a picture of them on the wine rack, throw darts at it and think about how smug you'll be in a month's time.

It can be really upsetting when people respond like this and it's important that you don't let their negativity compromise your success. Maybe this is just 'banter' for them, so let them know you're serious. They might reconsider and become your biggest supporter. If they persist in putting you down, I'd avoid this person for the next few weeks, and focus on the people who help and don't hinder your goals.

The Fact-Faker

This person must spend all their time on Google because whatever you've got to say they've got a fact that proves you wrong. They'll tell you that research says that a month off alcohol won't make a difference to your wellbeing (read it in a medical journal), wine is actually good for you (saw a TV programme about it), you're likely to binge for the rest of the year if you stop for a month (someone told them that it really does happen).

What to do: There's just no point arguing with the Fact-Faker, they'll always have a new set of stats to prove their point. Ignore them. Do your own research. Use the weekly check-in to monitor your progress and see how far you've come. You can become the living proof that their 'facts' are wrong!

To build you up (and for if you really lose your temper with the Fact-Faker and need something to throw back at them), here are some of the findings of research into Dry January by the University of Sussex. After one month dry . . .

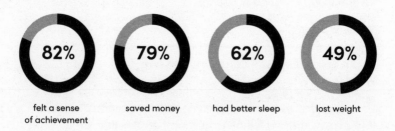

| 82% | 79% | 62% | 49% |
| felt a sense of achievement | saved money | had better sleep | lost weight |

The 'Why?'

This person challenges your reasons for going dry. They bombard you with questions and for every answer you give they've got a 'Yes, but . . . ' in reply. You can end up constantly justifying your actions to someone who doesn't really care – they just like a good argument.

A close relative of the 'Why?' is the Just Don't Get It. Their opening salvo usually consists of 'What do you want to do that for? You're not an alcoholic, are you?' They can't see the benefits and enjoy reiterating possible downsides.

What to do: You know what? You're not doing it for them. It doesn't matter what they think. You don't need them to agree, or even to get it. It's best not to ask their opinion, but – usually – if you tell them that you want their support, they'll rally round. Once they're fighting your corner, they're a good teammate to have.

The Saboteur

The Saboteur is a sneak. They outwardly offer support but secretly undermine your efforts. Sometimes they don't even know they're doing it, although perhaps that wide-eyed innocence is just an act. It might be your partner who brings home your favourite tipple on Friday night ('Oops, sorry – I forgot, shame to waste it, I can't drink it all myself') or the 'Go on, just one, I won't tell' mate. Either way, this person makes it easy for you to fall off the wagon.

What to do: Who do you know who might do this? Who's done it before with other challenges you've taken on?

If you can withstand their first couple of attacks they'll soon give up. Look at anyone who offers you alcohol suspiciously. Are they a saboteur? If you think they are, turn the tables on them: 'Sorry love, I'll just pour my half down the sink so that I'm not tempted.'

Use your weekly check-in to consider any sabotage attempts that may have happened during the week.

The Miserable Git

There's always someone who doesn't think it's a good idea, isn't there? It doesn't matter what the idea is, no good will come of it. Their glass is always half empty – and even more so when yours is full of a delicious alcohol-free alternative. No change is ever for the better and you're putting them out by wanting to complete your challenge. Basically, it's all about them. The Miserable Git isn't necessarily hostile, they can just be half-hearted in their response and useless in a crisis.

What to do: Start by reassuring them that this won't impact on them in any way. Don't try to sell them the idea; they'll see the changes in you soon enough.

The Green-Eyed Monster

The G-EM could be any of the above. Chances are, they think they'd struggle to do a month without a drink and your challenge is a threat. They don't want you to succeed because they don't have confidence in their own ability to go dry.

Alternatively, they get super competitive – you're going dry for a month, they'll do a year. You're doing it to feel better? They're raising money for tragically orphaned hedgehogs.

What to do: Don't take it personally. If someone's comments are worrying you then talk to them about it. They might not be aware that it's upsetting you. If nothing changes, you could probably do with keeping away from them for a while.

Hopefully, though, you'll come across plenty of positive, encouraging people instead.

Drew

'I found that if I was in a group of people, I was fearful of saying I didn't drink; like there was a stigma attached to it. But in the end it wasn't like that. People asked, "Oh yeah, why are you not drinking?" Not one person was judgemental or negative in any way. In fact, it brought out some very interesting conversations, with people saying, "Do you know what? I've been thinking about doing that as well." It was bizarrely cathartic and completely the opposite to what I was expecting, which was really empowering.'

—

4. THROUGHOUT THE MONTH

Here I want to give you a few more tried and tested tools to help you through the month.

Think about any month of your life. There are good months and bad months but mostly a mix of ups and downs – and the month you lay off the booze won't be any different. You need to give a little bit of your attention to it every day. That way, should an obstacle arise, you're already in the right mindset to deal with it.

MINDFULNESS

Mindfulness has become a bit of a buzz word, hasn't it? Everyone's gone mindfulness crazy. But at its core, it's just about paying attention to what's going on in your head and your body.

There's lots of evidence that practising mindfulness not only helps us to connect with what's really going on in our heads, but has benefits for our overall wellbeing. It allows us to become more in tune with our thoughts and emotions and this in turn helps us to recognise any unhelpful thoughts and stop them before they become intrusive.

When it comes to changing habits, mindfulness can help to build your resilience and stop you from slipping up without thinking about it. All of this is really handy if you sometimes absent-mindedly reach for a drink and don't even notice you're doing it.

→ Here are some simple exercises that you could try. If you've never done this kind of thing before, you might think it's a bit silly, or perhaps you just don't think it'll work. But I reckon the fact that you've got this far in the book means that you're up for trying some new stuff. So give it a go.

Every day

Here's a great mindfulness exercise that you can practise every day. Don't think you'll have time every day? You only need a minute or so for the following exercise.

Sit in a comfortable position on a chair with your hands resting on your lap and your feet touching the floor.

Close your eyes. Resist the urge to laugh.

Breathe deeply in and out, allowing your diaphragm and stomach to expand and relax with each breath.

Consciously relax each part of your body starting from the top of your head.

Move down to your face, jaw, neck and shoulders.

Relax your arms, hands and fingers; your back and stomach.

Relax your pelvis in your seat; your thighs, knees, calves and ankles.

Feel the ground through your feet and relax your heels, arches and toes.

If you notice your mind wandering away, just bring it back to focus on relaxing each part of your body.

Useful for:

Pausing between changing activities

Winding down at the end of the day

Stilling your mind during busy periods

Freaking out commuters on the number 50 bus

Tamal

'What I found especially good was to focus on the "now" and not get caught up worrying about things in the future that I have no control over.'

Week one

Repeat this exercise during the first week of your Try Dry challenge.

Every time you think about having an alcoholic drink, notice where you are, what you're doing, who you're with and how you feel about having the drink. Make a mental note and then carry on as before. Don't change what you do and (this is really important) don't have a go at yourself or put yourself down. You're trying to observe yourself with curiosity, not punish yourself.

Useful for:

Learning what thoughts and moods you associate with having a drink (see also the 'Fill the Gap' activity on page 78 and Chapter 6 on cravings)

Realising how often alcohol is mentioned on billboards, on TV and in magazines

Weeks two and three

During the second and third weeks of your challenge, take this exercise a little further. This will help you to recognise your self-sabotaging thoughts.

Pay attention to your thoughts. Every time you catch yourself thinking something negative about yourself, make a mental comment – 'Oh, I just put myself down,' or 'I brushed aside that compliment.' Don't try to change your thoughts, just notice them and move on. As with the last exercise, it's important not to judge yourself for these thoughts, just to notice that they are happening.

During the first weeks you may have trouble remembering to catch the thoughts. That's OK. When you remember that you've forgotten – don't give yourself a hard time about that either. As you practise, you will become more used to noticing and responding to your thoughts. For a while you may feel that you're thinking more negatively. Don't worry, this is normal, you're just becoming more aware.

Useful for:

Learning not to judge yourself for your thoughts

Practising connecting with your thoughts and feelings

Increasing awareness of your responses to others

Staying in the present moment

Ignoring bitchy comments on social media

Week four

The final part of this exercise, for week four of your challenge, is to smile when you notice one of these negative thoughts and say to yourself, 'That's not me.'

Useful for:

Choosing to divert negative thoughts before you become entangled with them

Feeling better about yourself

Really freaking out the commuters on the number 50 bus

Keeping yourself in the present

Do you find yourself going over old conversations or reliving past events? Do you daydream about the future or constantly practise future conversations that you probably won't have? Or does your mind keep wandering to drinks you'll have later, or after the month is over? Yeah – this is normal.

While it can be great to plan ahead, you're actually missing out on the here and now as you do so. If you notice yourself disappearing into the past or the future just say, 'Here and now, here and now,' to yourself to bring yourself back into the present.

As Master Oogway from *Kung Fu Panda* would say: 'Yesterday is history; tomorrow is a mystery; today is a gift, that's why it's called the present.' (He also said: 'Quit, don't quit. Noodles, don't noodles. You are too concerned with what was and what will be.' That is one wise tortoise.)

Useful for:

Letting go of unhelpful thoughts

Staying in the present moment

Impressing legendary, panda-shaped dragon warriors

Letting go of the day

OK, let's take it up a notch. This is a really, really useful exercise to help you get to sleep. If your mind races at night and you've been relying on booze to nod off, this one's for you. It works best if you listen to the words below when you're about to go to sleep.

'Listen?' I hear you say, 'How can I listen to it?'

Glad you asked. Record yourself reading the script below, slowly, and play it back at bedtime – simple! Better still, call up Tom Hardy and get him to record it for you.

If Tom Hardy isn't picking up and you don't have your record-o-matic (or smartphone) to hand, you can just imagine the warm golden ball moving up your body, relaxing and refreshing you as it goes. Again, no chuckling at the thought of golden balls, please. This is serious stuff. By the way, where it says pause, don't say pause. Just pause. Got it?

Lie on your back with your eyes closed. Breathe in slowly and breathe out slowly. Focus on the breath entering and leaving your body. (Pause.)

Imagine a warm ball of light hovering by your feet. You can feel the warmth of the ball on the soles of your feet and, as you feel it, your feet begin to relax. You can feel the ball moving slowly over your toes, pausing before it moves upwards to your ankles. Your feet are relaxed and warm. (Pause.)

The ball is moving slowly up your shins and the golden warmth penetrates to the backs of your calves through your bones, leaving your legs feeling totally relaxed. You can feel all tension leaving your muscles as the ball passes upwards to your knees. You can feel the gentle heat of the ball through your knees radiating upwards toward your thighs. (Pause.)

As the ball drifts over your thighs, the muscles let go and absorb the warmth from above. Your thighs and pelvis feel comfortable and relaxed, all tension released and the soothing ball passes higher and higher until it's over your stomach. (Pause.)

You can feel the ball, like a warm sun, floating over your torso, easing any aches and penetrating deep into your organs. It moves upward over your chest, resting for a few moments over your heart. Breathe in and breathe out, letting the warmth in with each breath. (Pause.)

The ball starts to expand so the warmth moves up towards your shoulders and out over your arms. You can feel your shoulders drop, relaxing as the warm glow moves out over your upper arms. The gentle heat expands further, warming your forearms and spreading its heat and light into your hands. You can feel the glow on the back of your hands and into your fingers, warming deeper and deeper into your arms, through the skin, into the bones. (Pause.)

The ball starts to move slowly up towards your neck, warming your chin and jaw and spreading relaxation through your neck muscles and into your face. (Pause.)

The ball creeps upwards, radiating warm light onto your face. You can feel its touch on your cheeks and eyelids, warming your ears and forehead. You feel your head relaxing as the ball warms through you. (Pause.)

The ball starts to move away over the top of your head. You feel a slight pull as all the cares and worries of the day start to drift out of your head and into the ball. They become absorbed into the warm ball of light and disappear. (Pause.)

The ball starts to recede, carrying your worries away, leaving you warm in your core and in your limbs and in your body and in your head. You are completely relaxed and ready for sleep.

Useful for:

Learning to sleep naturally, without the aid of alcohol

Relaxing both mind and body

If you find it hard to be mindful because as soon as you pause for a minute worries, shopping lists and other random thoughts pop into your head, that just means you're normal. It's natural to find your mind drifting away at first. The point is not to make these thoughts go away, but rather to become aware of them and let them pass by, without needing to linger over them or judge them or yourself.

The more you practise the easier it becomes. Most of us find it hard to remember to do this regularly at first, so I recommend downloading a mindfulness app too. There are some app suggestions in the resources section at the back of the book.

Being mindful is about releasing stress and focusing on your senses, rather than just your thoughts. If you're feeling particularly low and mindfulness doesn't seem to help you to relax, have a chat with your GP. You can also complete a useful mood self-assessment questionnaire on the NHS website.

FOOD GLORIOUS FOOD

Now that your inner peace is taken care of, what about the rest of your insides? Do you eat well? Hope so, because there's no point getting all 'clean on the inside' booze-wise if you're still eating 15 kebabs and 84 chocolate bars a day.

Ever looked on the back of your favourite tipple for the nutritional values? They're not there. Why do you think that is?

If you've been forgoing meals to use your recommended daily calories on booze, sure, you'll get lots of energy because alcohol is full of sugary carbs. But you won't get any of the protein, fats, vitamins or minerals that you need – that's why it's known as 'empty energy'. And no, wine and cider do not count as one of your five-a-day, just because they're made from fruits. Chugging a hoppy beer doesn't give you one portion of wholemeal grains, either. Want some of those antioxidants that are rumoured to be in red wine? Er, just eat red grapes!

Did you know that drinking can deplete your body of several different nutrients? In particular, B vitamins are hard for your liver to store when you drink. B vitamins are fabulous little micronutrients that raise your mood and improve your memory. Who doesn't want brighter moods and a better memory? More than that – they're actually essential to the function of your brain.

In fact, alcohol reduces your body's ability to absorb and use most of the lovely vitamins we need for good health, including vitamin C and much of the rest of the alphabet.

There you have it. Just taking a month off the grog will help your body to get more nourishment from whatever it is that you do eat. Why not combine that with treating your new-found tastebuds (yes, they work better too) by checking out new restaurants, seasonal fruits and other edible delights during your dry adventure?

Some Try Dryers have reported that they tend to eat more when they lay off the booze; especially sweet stuff. Others say that they find it easier to control their eating without the booze demon sitting on their shoulder urging them to snaffle a packet of salt-and-vinegar before bed. Either way, taking a little time to think about your nutrition for the month will help you make the most of your journey. But definitely don't beat yourself up too much about food during this month. Stay focused on winning that alcohol challenge you've set yourself. If you find your eating habits changing, perhaps just go with it for now (within reason).

TREAT YO'SELF

Ever use alcohol as a reward? Yeah, I know the feeling. You've had a hard day and a nice cold beer/glass of Cab Sav/Babycham would go down nicely. After all, you deserve it.

So what will you do during your dry month?

Well, just because you're not drinking doesn't mean you can't treat yourself – you just need to change the treat. Planning a little something for each evening so you've got something to look forward to will help to beat the midweek blues and keep you on track. In the immortal words of Donna from *Parks and Rec*: 'Treat yo'self!'

Here are a few ideas:

- Hot bath with scented candles

- Chocolate

- Trip to the gym

- No social media for an hour whilst reading a magazine/novel/birdwatching guide/literally anything that isn't Facebook

- Playing guitar

- Face mask, pedicure

- Chocolate

- Getting a takeaway instead of cooking

- Cooking instead of nuking something from the freezer

- Throwing darts at a picture of your boss

- Chocolate. OK, enough of the chocolate – I think we had both better go back to the previous page about nutrition and think of something else

- Bike ride

- Midweek film night

- Evening walk

- Horse riding (as you do)

- Hour on Xbox/PlayStation/games console of your choice

Write your own list of treats. Remember, cleaning the car just because you've now got bags of energy on Saturday morning is definitely not a treat. Your treat has to be something genuinely pleasurable. You should be sipping a latte somewhere, or browsing antique shops, or strolling through the park, or re-enacting the battle of Naseby with 500 or so of your closest friends.

FILL THE GAP

→ If it's not as a treat, why do you drink? We all have our reasons but most of us don't take the time to work out what role alcohol plays in our life. Look at the table over the page – what are your reasons for drinking? Once you've got them ticked, is there anything else you could do to get a similar effect?

What you're trying to do here is find something positive to fill the role that alcohol plays in your life. That way you haven't lost something; you've replaced it.

If you tick all of them – believe me, life will get a whole lot more interesting when you stop using alcohol as your default solution for everything.

Why I have a drink	✔	Other things I can do instead
To relax		
To give me confidence		
Because I like the taste		
To celebrate		
Because I'm angry		
Because my partner is drinking		
It's just habit		
To relieve boredom		
For company		
To feel better		
To help me sleep		
To relieve stress		
It's expected of me		
To block out worries		
Because I'm upset		
It makes me feel sociable		
Because I have a craving		
Other reason:		
Other reason:		

DRY DIARY

Making time every day – even just a couple of minutes – to remind yourself of why you're doing this and how far you've come will really help you to see it through to the end. Some people find it helpful to keep a Dry Diary (Dryary?). Record what's new, what's different, what's better every day, what you're up to now you're not drinking. You can look back at previous entries and see just how far you've come. It'll help you to figure out your reasons for drinking and it can help with this whole mindfulness thing I keep banging on about.

Or, if you like to share, why not blog about your experiences, or share updates via social media? This might help to inspire your friends and family or just keep you thinking about your Try Dry goals.

→ If you're not into a daily diary or blogging, then I would really recommend the simple weekly check-in below. It could just make the difference between a successful dry month and an unsuccessful one, especially where success for you involves changing your drinking once your dry month is done.

Weekly check-in

This week my mood is:

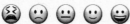

This week my happiness rating is:

1   2   3   4   5   6   7   8   9   10

This week my energy levels are:

1   2   3   4   5   6   7   8   9   10

My sleep over the last week has been:

1   2   3   4   5   6   7   8   9   10

What I've found challenging about the week:

What I've found most rewarding about the week:

What I'm most proud of:

What I've learned:

What's been most useful to me:

What I'll do differently next week:

What my plan is for next week:

Lily

'Previously I kept getting the feeling that there was a word I needed to use, but I couldn't quite retrieve it from my brain. At the end of Dry January the words come more easily . . . My brain has cleared!'

—

Cadence

'When people say their skin and their hair become amazing you think, "Oh really?" But they do, they really do.'

—

5. BRAIN AND BODY

Back in 2013, Rajiv Jalan, a liver specialist at the Institute for Liver and Digestive Health at University College London Medical School – yep, that's a real thing – teamed up with a group of staff from the *New Scientist* to see what effect just a month off alcohol could have on liver health.[*] He got really excited about the results. He noted liver fat reductions of up to 20 per cent and an average drop in blood glucose levels of 16 per cent. In other words, just four weeks off the booze may reduce risks of liver disease and diabetes. Not bad, eh?

Hopefully you're convinced of the rewards of a dry month by now and keen to experience them for yourself, but if you need any more persuading then here's the science bit, where we tell you exactly what's going on in that incredible body of yours with and without a drink.

Me: I heard that red wine is good for you.

Myself: Wayyy! Excellent news. Crack open the Chateauneuf, I'm feeling a bit peaky.

Dr I: Not so fast. According to the latest guidelines, we should be drinking less not more.

Myself: Yeah, but red wine's OK – it's got antioxidants!

Dr I: True, but it's also got alcohol, which makes it a mixed blessing. As soon as you go over a small amount of alcohol per week, your risk starts to increase – so if you think you can let loose

---

[*] Coghlan, A., 2013, 'Our liver vacation: Is a dry January really worth it?', *New Scientist* 2, 950.

on the red wine and your heart will benefit, you're wrong. And you can get more of those antioxidants from red grapes, anyway . . .

Me: First point to Dr I.

Myself: Dammit.

WHAT HAPPENS WHEN YOU DRINK

At the first glug	Did you know that alcohol isn't digested? It's absorbed. The difference is that it doesn't wait until it reaches your intestine to start working its way into your bloodstream. From the moment you ingest it, alcohol starts to make its way around your body.
2 minutes	Once in the stomach, about 20 per cent is absorbed. The rest carries on to your small intestine where it passes into the bloodstream. If the stomach is empty, it will travel to the intestines more quickly. This is why we're often told not to drink on an empty stomach as it makes us feel the effects more quickly. Watch out though, this doesn't mean that having a Big Mac before a bender will act as a super-shield to protect your body from the effects.
5 minutes	By this time the booze has reached your brain. Once there it disrupts chemical messages in different regions causing the range of effects that we know and love . . . and those we're not so keen on. Everything from conscious actions like movement and thought to automatic functions like breathing and temperature control are affected. Essentially, we become less good at doing lots of stuff. We're also getting dehydrated. And repeated heavy drinking over a long period can cause permanent damage to our neurons, the message carriers in our brains, leading to problems with memory, coordination and thinking.

30 minutes	It takes about this long for the alcohol to be absorbed and to be circulating through your bloodstream. It then passes to the liver for elimination. In about 30 minutes your blood alcohol concentration is starting to peak and that tipsy feeling has kicked in. As alcohol is a muscle relaxant, the muscular ring at the bottom of your oesophagus can get a bit too chilled and allow stomach acid through, causing acid reflux or heartburn.
60 minutes	It takes an hour for one unit of alcohol to be broken down by your liver. Your liver can't work any faster than this (no matter how much coffee or water you drink) so if you consume more than one unit of alcohol in an hour, the rest will have to take a ticket and wait its turn in the bloodstream. Up to about 10 per cent of the alcohol is breathed out through your lungs (hence breathalysers) and the rest is broken down into carbon dioxide and water, which you will be excreting for the rest of the evening.
2 hours	If we continue to drink during this time we can expect to experience a range of psychological effects such as euphoria, sociability, paranoia, increased aggression and sudden mood swings. Physical effects are likely to include vomiting, poor coordination and terrible dancing. Our social sensibilities have become much weaker, which is why we don't notice we're hogging the karaoke machine.
Up to 6 hours	After four or more drinks your risk of injury is increased for about six hours as high levels of blood alcohol disrupt your coordination and thought processes. During this time you tend to be more clumsy or forgetful. You may fall asleep quickly, but it's unlikely to be particularly restful sleep.
Up to about 10 hours	Sleep is disturbed for a number of reasons, including the blocking of REM sleep (the bit where you dream), interruption to your circadian rhythm (normal day/night cycles), the diuretic effect (er, you know, extra trips to the bathroom), relaxation of throat muscles (snoring) and poor temperature control (sweating).

Up to about 18 hours	You're likely to have a lower mood because of the depletion of a chemical called dopamine in the brain, the loss of important minerals and reduced glycogen, which makes blood sugar levels drop.

Great. So now we know what it is that our body is giving up for a few weeks. But how does *not* drinking impact on our body and brain? Let's take a stroll through a month without a drink and explore what we can expect to see as the days roll by. Everyone is different, of course – results will vary. Don't sit up waiting for the appearance of each new effect on the stroke of midnight.

Some benefits will be more obvious than others, but here's a good tip: ask your nearest and dearest what they've spotted. They might notice changes that you've missed. The first time my long-suffering better half took a dry month he complained that it had no effect at all until I pointed out that:

- He was getting out of bed on the first alarm rather than pressing snooze several times.

- He'd started singing in the shower.

- He wasn't snoring.

- He spent a lot less time frantically rushing round the house yelling: 'Where are my keys? Have you seen my wallet? What did I do with my phone?'

- By the end of the month he was 7lbs lighter and annoyingly energetic at the weekend.

Drew

'The thing that made me go "Wow" was how people proactively came up to me and said, "You look really good. What have you done? What have you changed?" To the point where I thought, "Blimey, I must have looked really ropey."'

A QUICK GUIDE TO YOUR DRY MONTH

DAYS 1–3

Assuming you don't spend the night before you start your challenge trying to remove all booze from the house by drinking it, the first 24 hours will see your body eliminating alcohol from your system at the rate of one unit per hour (after the first half hour, when it's just absorbing, not processing). You probably won't feel any different. After all, most of us regularly manage a day without drinking. Use one of the drink tracker apps or the oh-so-much-fun calculation on page 28 to work out how many units you drink in a typical evening and you'll be able to pinpoint pretty accurately when the booze has left the building.

Hello, grumpy! You may feel a bit under the weather as dopamine, a mood-enhancing chemical produced in the brain, is still depleted and your body is replacing glycogen and minerals. If you're feeling sluggish and low, and find yourself snapping at everyone, just remember that this will only last a few days at most and the good stuff is just around the corner.

You may find that it takes a while to drop off to sleep during the first week. Without the soporific effect of booze to knock us out, we don't plummet into unconsciousness quite so quickly. It's tempting to have a drink to get you off to sleep, but then you'd be back to square one.

Make sure you've got a good sleep hygiene routine – try to go to bed at the same time each night. Don't eat just before bedtime and limit screen time, going completely screen-free for the hour or so before bed. Milky drinks, warm baths, soothing music, reading *Ulysses* – you might need to try a few things before you hit on your best sleep aids.

Me: Day 3. Why do I feel so crap? I'm achy, tired and miserable. I'm not sleeping and my head wants to explode.

Myself: We knew this would happen.

Dr I: Remember that time we gave up coffee?

Me: Vaguely. I mainly remember the pounding head and extreme sleepiness.

Myself: We told you that was a bad idea too, but no one listens to us.

Dr I: Don't worry, that passed, didn't it? This is just our body getting rid of all the toxins it's been storing. Once they're out of the way we'll feel better.

Me: When? We need a timescale.

Myself: As soon as we have a drink.

Dr I: Then we'd have to start this all over again. Nearly there, give it 72 hours and we'll be on top of the world.

Me: Promise?

Dr I: Promise.

Myself: Creep.

DAYS 4–7

Hopefully you're feeling much better by now. All of your body's systems are back to their usual working levels. You may find that you have more energy and better concentration. Even if you toss and turn a bit at first, when you do drop off you'll get better-quality sleep and probably wake feeling more refreshed the next day. You may notice that you're not getting up for the 3 a.m. wee, too, which is a nice bonus.

Some people experience very vivid dreams around this time. This could be down to increased rapid eye movement (REM) sleep. REM is the stage of sleep during which we dream. When we drink, REM sleep is suppressed, which is why we're still so tired the next day, even after an eight-hour slumber. A few days off the booze and – hey presto!

These dreams are nothing to worry about but some people do report that they're the craziest, scariest or most outlandish and lucid dreams they've ever had. Popcorn, anyone?

DAYS 8–10

If you've been suffering from acid reflux, a burning sensation in the throat also known as heartburn, you should be noticing a reduction by now.

You may find that you have more energy and your thinking is clearer, too. Lots of people describe this as 'the fog lifting'. You may find it easier to get up in the mornings and you'll be less prone to mood swings.

By this time you've completed your first sober weekend – well done! How did you find it? If you're typically a weekend drinker, it might have been a bit of a novelty to wake up without feeling the effects of last night. Hopefully you came up with some alternative activities so you weren't tempted by the end of the work week. Did you learn anything from spending a weekend sober? What are you going to plan for next weekend? Check out chapters 9 and 10 for activity ideas.

DAYS 11–14

Are you drinking more water? Now that you've been off alcohol for nearly two weeks, you may notice that you're thirstier. It's not that you need more fluids than normal, just that you're more in tune with just how much you do need. Stay hydrated – it's a big help for one of the lovely effects that may be coming up in week four.

How's your exercise routine going? Alcohol is a muscle relaxant so regular drinking can reduce muscle development. Now you're dry, all that hard work you put in at the gym (ahem) might finally start paying off. If you're not a regular exerciser but have been thinking about giving it a go, there couldn't be a better time.

DAYS 15–21

Alongside your new svelte physique from all that exercise, you may be noticing the pounds dropping off too. As the average pint can rack up 200+ calories and a large glass of wine about the same it's easy to see why you might find your waistband loosening after a couple of weeks.

One study showed that men are likely to eat more calories but less fruit and milk, while women eat more fat on days when they drink.[*] Research has also found that you're likely to eat more during a meal if you've had alcohol first.[†]

On the other hand, if you find that you're not dropping any weight, it could be because alcohol, like sugar, initially boosts the levels of happy chemicals in your brain. So, when you stop drinking, you may start to crave sugar and find you're snacking a lot more. Don't worry, that's normal. If you're not happy with your new sweet tooth, though, check out Chapter 6 on beating cravings.

By now, you might also start to notice improvements in your memory, particularly your short-term memory. You might find that you can retain information for longer, you're less forgetful or that you're more able to focus your attention.

---

[*] Breslow, R. A., et al, 2013, 'Diets of drinkers on drinking and nondrinking days: NHANES 2003-2008', *American Journal of Clinical Nutrition* 97(5), 1068–75.
[†] Eiller, J. A., et al, 2015, 'The apéritif effect: Alcohol's effects on the brain's response to food aromas in women', *Obesity Society Journal* 23(7), 1386-93.

DAYS 22-28

Another lovely side effect of no booze might start to appear around this time: your skin starting to look amazing. Alcohol reduces the production of anti-diuretic hormone, so you lose water and sodium more quickly. A low tissue water content, courtesy of your daily tipple, is the sworn enemy of soft, plump, peachy skin. Booze is also one of the big triggers for rosacea, or facial redness. As if that wasn't enough, a few weeks off the sauce should see the size of facial pores diminish too.

If you've got high blood pressure, there's a good chance it'll start to come down by the end of your challenge. Research has found that just four weeks without a drink can be enough to start lowering both blood pressure and heart rate.[*]

Your risk of type 2 diabetes has already started to reduce (in one study insulin resistance came down by an average of 28 per cent) and your cholesterol levels should be starting to lower.

But what about your liver? Your poor old liver has to process booze into waste products along with the other 500 or so tasks it performs in your body. So giving it a little holiday means that it can focus on its other jobs. One research study found that just four weeks without a drink can substantially reduce liver 'stiffness'.[†] Brilliant! Who wants a stiff liver?! (This stiffness is an early sign of liver disease, in case you were wondering.)

And how about number twos? If you've been experiencing bloating, wind and either diarrhoea or constipation, you've probably noticed a reduction in symptoms by now. Relief all round.

---

[*]   Teresa Aguilera, M., de la Sierra, A., Coca, Antonio, Estruch, Ramon, Fernández-Solà, Joaquim, Urbano-Márquez, A., 1999, 'Effect of alcohol abstinence on blood pressure: Assessment by 24-Hour ambulatory blood pressure monitoring', *Hypertension* 33, 653-7.
[†]   Mehta, G., et al., 2015, 'Short term abstinence from alcohol improves insulin resistance and fatty liver phenotype in moderate drinkers', *Hepatology* 62(1), 267A.

Me: Is it true that after giving up drinking for a month, I'm much more likely to hit the bottle hard and undo all that good work?

Myself: My point exactly. Why go through all this when we're only going to make things worse by getting mullered for the next year anyway?

Dr I: Research shows—

Myself: Shut up about bloody research!

Dr I: As we were saying, research shows that we're less likely to increase our drinking. In fact we're likely still to be drinking less harmfully six months later, drinking on fewer days, and finding it easier to say no to a drink.

Me: Another slam dunk for Dr I.

AFTER 28 DAYS

Congratulations! Your risk of developing certain cancers, including two of the most common worldwide – breast and colorectal – is diminishing. According to a 2018 report in the *Lancet*, by reducing your drinking, you also reduce your risk of strokes, heart disease and hypertensive disease and could increase your life expectancy.[*]

You have also reduced your tolerance to alcohol so if you start drinking again you won't be able to drink as much as before. Cheap date, in other words. Watch out for this, it can take you by surprise just how quickly your body has re-adapted to not knocking back the booze.

---

[*] Wood, A. M., et al., 2018, 'Risk thresholds for alcohol consumption: Combined analysis of individual-participant data for 599,912 current drinkers in 83 prospective studies', *Lancet* 391(10 129), 1513–23.

Booze suppresses your body's immune system, so when you're free and clear of it for a few weeks you'll notice that you are less likely to succumb to every little cold virus that hits the office, and even if you do come down with something, your recovery time will be reduced. There. Hope you're feeling better already.

Oi – where are my Try Dry benefits?

Some people will experience these benefits at different times, or not at all. This can be down to how much you were drinking before, other lifestyle changes (if you're ditching your nightcap for an espresso, you're not likely to have better sleep) or just the quirks of your particular body.

That doesn't mean your month off isn't doing you good, and it doesn't mean you won't feel better over the longer term – so don't give up if you're not experiencing these effects exactly as they're laid out above. And keep an eye out for benefits I don't mention!

MORE FUN FACTS ABOUT ALCOHOL AND YOU
IF YOU'RE UNDER 18

How come you're reading this book?

You're still growing. So filling your body with a substance with a lot of nasty side effects is not the best move. Many of us adults have been setting a bad example, but do yourself a favour and be better than us!

If you're drinking more than you think you should, it's worth having a chat with someone about it. You might think your parents are a no-go, but they could actually be the best people to talk to. Failing that, your GP is a good place to start and will keep everything confidential, or use the local services directory on the Alcohol Change UK website.

18-29

Your brain is still developing until your mid-20s, especially your pre-frontal cortex – which is why you're probably more impulsive than you will be when you're older. Research suggests heavy drinking at this age can have long-term effects on this development. You may also be starting to set drinking habits that can last a lifetime.

30-39

By now your brain and body have matured but if you're still drinking like you did in your student days, you've probably noticed that the hangovers last longer and hit you harder than a decade ago. This is down to both the normal ageing process and the fact that your tolerance and therefore your drinking, have inched up over the years. Your thirties are often when you consider starting a family and, believe me, simultaneously taking care of a toddler and a hangover is not ideal. It's a good plan to get a handle on your drinking habits before contemplating parenthood.

40-50

By this age, many of us have growing families, responsibilities, jobs, homes etc., and alcohol may just be one of those habits that we've picked up along the way without really thinking about it. But this is the age at which many alcohol-specific deaths peak, such as liver disease.* Literally, a sobering thought.

*   Public Health England, 15 September 2017, 'The 2nd Atlas of Variation in risk factors and healthcare for liver disease in England', retrieved from www.england.nhs.uk.

IF YOU'RE OVER 50

As you mature, you may find that you just *can't* drink as much as you used to, but you are more likely to be drinking every day than your younger counterparts.

As we age, our bodies change on the inside, as well as the inevitable increase in wrinkles on the outside. We start to lose muscle and gain fat and are less able to break down alcohol so effectively. In other words, our bodies become more sensitive to its effects.

You'll probably find that, as part of the normal ageing process, your reactions start to slow, your memory is not as sharp as it used to be and you can be a little unsteady on your feet – and that's before you hit the tequila. Alcohol can impair all of these functions further.

You're also more likely to be taking medication for some other ailment that you shouldn't combine with alcohol. Grab a magnifying glass and read the little leaflet that comes with your medication – if it advises no booze, best to keep off the drink until you finish the meds.

Long-term heavy drinking can also cause dementia.[*]

IF YOU'RE FEMALE

Sorry, ladies. It's not good news. On the whole, women are much more at risk from the negative aspects of alcohol than men. We've got a higher body fat and lower water percentage in our bodies than men (as if we needed reminding) and this means that booze is more concentrated as it travels round our body. We also have less of the liver enzyme that breaks alcohol down from a toxic substance to harmless carbon dioxide and

---

[*]   Pollock, B. G., et al., 2018, 'Contribution of alcohol use disorders to the burden of dementia in France 2008–13: A nationwide retrospective cohort study', *Lancet Public Health* 3(3), e124–e132.

water. The upshot is that it takes less alcohol for us to feel drunk and causes more long-term harm at lower levels of drinking.

As if that wasn't bad enough, drinking can disrupt menstruation, and you can become intoxicated more rapidly in the days before your period. Regular heavy drinking can also reduce fertility.* Not recommended as a form of contraception, though.

Drinking during pregnancy isn't recommended either. While we don't know exactly how much alcohol it takes to harm a foetus, we do know that the more you drink, the higher the risk to both mother and baby. Alcohol can cause a number of birth defects, known collectively as foetal alcohol spectrum disorders. So if you're planning to become pregnant it's safer to abstain.

By the time you enter peri-menopause in your late 40s or 50s, there's a whole new factor to consider – alcohol seems to exacerbate hot flushes, night sweats and mood swings. And then, just to top it off, drinking increases your risk of breast cancer. The highest breast cancer risk is for post-menopausal women.[†]

IF YOU'RE MALE

If you thought you were going to get off lightly because you're a bloke, think again. OK, you may not have to worry about all that hormonal stuff but there's definitely a bunch of risks with your name on them – increased blood pressure, high cholesterol, obesity, and coronary heart disease, to name just a few.

And to add insult to injury, here are two words guaranteed to get your attention: erectile dysfunction. It may take more alcohol to raise your blood alcohol content to dangerous levels than it does for women, but brewer's droop doesn't care. As Shakespeare once said, 'It provokes the desire, but it takes away

---

*   Mikkelsen, E. M., et al., 2016, 'Alcohol consumption and fecundability: Prospective Danish cohort study', *British Medical Journal* 354:i4262.
†   World Breast Cancer Research Fund, Breast Cancer 2017 Report.

the performance.' Nicely put, Will. That's *Macbeth*, Act 2, Scene 3, in case you were wondering.

If you do manage to, er, raise the flag, so to speak, you might still be out of luck, fertility-wise. So if you're planning a baby, best to keep that drinking well under control.

WEEKLY BINGE VS DAILY DABBLE

This is a longstanding debate. Which is worse for your health – daily drinking or weekly binges? Ah, if only it were as simple as that. But let's imagine two people drinking the same number of units each week, but one goes for a daily 250ml glass of wine (three units) and the other drinks seven glasses (that's two-and-a-third bottles, or 21 units) in one night. Who is better off?

Research suggests that daily drinkers are more prone to liver disease because they don't take time off to let the liver have a bit of a rest, but bingers are often exposed to risks that daily drinkers are not.[*] There are serious safety risks associated with binge drinking as your coordination, judgement and consciousness begin to fail. Drowning after falling into water is another serious risk.

I once explained to a group of teenagers that inhaling his own vomit after a binge was the way we lost the late, great Jimi Hendrix. 'Who's that?' asked one of the group. 'He's that snooker player,' replied another.

The Chief Medical Officers in the UK recommend a maximum of 14 units a week for adults, spread throughout the week and with several days off.

---

[*]   Hatton, J., Burton, A., Nash, H., Munn, E., Burgoyne, L. & Sheron, N., 2009, 'Drinking patterns, dependency and life-time drinking history in alcohol-related liver disease', *Addiction* 104, 587-592.

ALCOHOL AND MEDICATION

There are three sorts of reaction that alcohol may have when mixed with other substances. And I don't just mean medicines here, I'm talking about illegal drugs too.

Depending on the medication or drug, alcohol may:

- Increase the blood level of a drug, or vice versa

- Alter the action of the other drug in the body

- Combine to make a completely different and more toxic substance

Drinking while taking medicine can have serious consequences so it's always best to read the leaflet carefully and check with your pharmacist if you're unsure.

ALCOHOL AND SPORT

You'd think that these two go together like bacon and eggs, especially if you check out all the alcohol companies sponsoring and advertising through sport, right? But when it comes to actually *playing* sports, drinking can really hamper performance. If you don't believe me, try doing a half marathon with a hangover. Incidentally, people also report that watching sport is much more enjoyable when you can actually follow the game.

Drinking is likely to dehydrate your body and lower your blood glucose levels, neither of which make for a personal best on the track; not to mention its effect on coordination and concentration. So, you should probably be resting the morning after the night before, not lifting weights or shakin' your Zumba stuff. And no, you cannot 'run off' alcohol or sweat it out.

If you do decide to work on your fitness while a bit the worse for wear, remember to drink plenty of water and take it easy – your risk of injury is increased and your recovery time will be longer.

In the longer term, drinking can hamper your muscle development and frustrate efforts to lose weight so it's best to keep it as an occasional treat if you want to reach your fitness goals.

Me: Why do we get hangovers?

Myself: Because we're utter lightweights and can't hold our booze?

Dr I: There are lots of factors that make us feel ill after drinking – dehydration, poor sleep, acid reflux, loss of minerals such as magnesium and sodium.

Me: So what can we do about it?

Myself: Oooh, we know this one – hair of the dog!

Dr I: Actually, that will instantly make us feel better but it's a bad idea.

Me: Sounds pretty good actually, I'm with Myself for once.

Myself: Yeah, Dr I, take that!

Dr I: More grog will just delay the inevitable – what goes up must come down, so by avoiding the Sunday-morning hangover we're literally giving ourselves a bigger headache later. Why not try plenty of fluids, a duvet day and some nice scrambled eggs instead?

Me: Sorry, Myself, that's a much better plan.

(Anybody noticed yet that if you say Dr I quickly it actually sounds like Dry? Almost like I planned it that way.)

YOUR TRY DRY HEALTH DIARY

→ Use the diaries on the next pages to record how you feel throughout your challenge.

Day 1

	😣	🙁	😐	🙂	😃
My sleep					
My mood					
My energy					
Aches and pains					
Stress					
Comments					

Day 8

	😣	🙁	😐	🙂	😃
My sleep					
My mood					
My energy					
Aches and pains					
Stress					
Comments					

Day 15

	😫	🙁	😐	🙂	😄
My sleep					
My mood					
My energy					
Aches and pains					
Stress					
Comments					

Day 22

	😫	🙁	😐	🙂	😄
My sleep					
My mood					
My energy					
Aches and pains					
Stress					
Comments					

Day 29

	😫	😟	😐	🙂	😄
My sleep					
My mood					
My energy					
Aches and pains					
Stress					
Comments					

6. CRAVINGS

After the initial high of the first few days off the booze, when the first flush of motivation starts to wear thin, you might start to crave a drink.

Before you begin to panic and check yourself into celebrity rehab, STOP! Don't worry, this doesn't mean you've got 'a problem'. It's a normal reaction to change. It's so normal, in fact, that we've included a cravings journal in this book. This is for you to fill in every time you get a craving. It's not meant for every time the thought pops into your head: 'Oh, a drink would be nice right now.' The cravings journal is for you to record just those unexpected, powerful urges to seek out a drink. Flip to the end of this chapter to check it out.

Cravings can be crushing. At first we're brimming with enthu-siasm and confidence, staying dry, feeling proud, and then, at some point, it dawns on us that it's just the normal daily grind but with something missing. If drinking has formed part of your routine for years, even decades, then of course you're going to find yourself wanting to reach for it at some point in the month. But fear not. If you can recognise a craving for what it is and have a plan in place, even the most dogged of cravings can be overcome.

Interestingly, cravings are often not about the booze itself, but about a particular moment, trigger or emotion. If you've completed the 'Fill the Gap' activity in Chapter 4 you might have already worked this out. When we're stressed or upset or bored, we seek comfort. That's natural, and if alcohol has been there for us through the hard times, then, bingo, that's what we think we want when the going gets tough.

The point is, the association with alcohol becomes just that: an association. If we can replace it with something else, then we can get through our tougher life moments *and* avoid the downsides that come with alcohol. Nowadays, personally, I head straight for the lemon drizzle or, at a push, the chocolate mini rolls.

SO WHAT EXACTLY IS A CRAVING?

Wanting a drink and having a craving are different things. If you just want a drink it's easy to make the conscious decision to do something else. A craving, however, can be a powerful beastie, all fangs and claws, and once it gets a grip on you it can feel nigh on impossible to wrench yourself free from its clutches. Think I'm exaggerating? Well, maybe a little, but it can overwhelm you, especially if your defences are low because you're having a bad day or you're feeling under the weather. At times it can feel as though you have no choice but to give in.

Andrew

'I was on the way home from work and I was thinking I could really murder a drink. There was a real need, a real craving. It was hugely helpful to have that normalised for me; that what I was going through was a craving, and most of us have them. It helped to strengthen my resolve.'

The thing is, we often get these cravings but don't think of them as such because we Just. Have. A. Drink. 'Oh look, I really want a drink. OK, so I'll have a drink. Mmm, nice drink.' Job done.

It's not until we have a reason *not* to pick up a glass that it becomes apparent that we've got a craving. So basically we often have cravings for things but we don't notice because we have access to the thing we crave. There's something about being told you can't have something, even when you're the one doing the telling, that makes you want it all the more.

There's research to suggest that cravings are most likely to surface when you are least confident in your ability to resist a drink. Typical.

Not all cravings are the same. They vary in intensity and length and, over time, as new pathways are formed in your brain, they start to diminish.

CRAVING WITHOUT CAVING

Think your cravings are insurmountable? Imagine this: you get a craving for a pint of best halfway through delivering a presentation to colleagues on widgets and whatsits, or in the middle of a cardio set at the gym. Do you rush out of the room, intent on tracking down said pint? Pushing petrified passers-by out of the way in your haste to sate your unquenchable beer need? No? (Please say no.) Of course not. You brush the thought aside and get on with what you were doing.

So, that tells us that when the craving is inconvenient or the reason for not giving in is important enough, that wicked little craving loses its potency. See, cravings can be overcome.

Don't believe me? Here's an activity for you. Find an ex-smoker, preferably someone who stopped more than a year ago, and ask them about cravings. They're sure to tell you that these were at their worst in the first few weeks after they stopped and that different things, people or situations triggered a desire to smoke. Now ask how they overcame their cravings. You can repeat this with every ex-smoker you can find; they'll all have had different strategies for not lighting up.

Here are five things that it will help to know:

1. If something else is more important, your craving will diminish.

2. Distraction works.

3. The bigger the craving, the more amazing you'll feel when you beat it.

4. Cravings don't last for ever.

5. Overcoming cravings is one of the biggest tasks you need to accomplish when going dry for a month – don't shirk this task, embrace it!

So, the good news is that you **can** overcome any craving, and the not-so-good news is that you're going to have to figure out for yourself what works for you. Luckily, there are a few suggestions in this chapter. Read on!

Deb

'My mum and sister came to visit. I got so angry. They would have their glass of wine and I wanted to give in. I just stuck with my kombucha. I remember it was tense and I was just recognising the physical irritation of not drinking.'

Two craving tales by Me, Myself and I

Scenario 1

Me: Our first time out without a drink; we *will* be OK, won't we?

Myself: Of course we will, unless someone talks to us, of course – then we'll crumble like a biscuit.

I: Practise our breathing, it'll help. Smile, everyone looks friendly.

Me: OK, bit more relaxed now.

Myself: Wow, this party rocks, everyone is drinking, having fun. Love it.

Me: I'm the only one without a glass of wine.

Myself: We're fine! Except . . . is that Merlot? It is! Our favourite!

I: Don't look! Don't look! Don't look!

Me: I can't help it, look at the way it sits invitingly in the glass.

Myself: Yeah, full body, legs, swirly in the glass. We always feel so much more relaxed at parties when we've had some.

I: Don't look! Don't look! Don't look!

Me: But I want it, I really want it. Please can I have it?

Myself: Shouldn't really but . . . the party will be ruined if we're sitting here thinking about it all night.

I: Mustn't. Look. Must. Walk. Away. Can't. Move.

Me: I can smell it, all fruity and velvety. It's in my head, I can't take much more of this.

Myself: True. You can't. We're just not good at not

drinking are we? Might as well have a glass. Let's face it, we'll feel better if we do and worse if we don't. No-brainer.

I: Nooooo!

Scenario 2

Me: Our first time without a drink; we *will* be OK, won't we?

I: Of course we will, I've locked Myself in the bathroom.

Me: Oh look, Merlot. Our favourite. That'd help us to relax.

I: Yes, but it wouldn't be us, it'd be the Merlot mingling. Tell you what, you know Stacey – why not go and chat to her?

Me: What if she blanks us?

I: What if she doesn't? What have we got to lose? If we stick around here we'll just stare at the Merlot all night.

Me: OK, I'll give it a try.

10 minutes later

Me: Stacey is so funny.

I: I know. That joke about the vicar in the sauna was hilarious. So glad we had that chat.

Me: I didn't even realise she wasn't drinking until she asked for that tonic water.

I: Yeah, she was so happy there was someone else not knocking back the wine. Who shall we talk to now?

TACTICS FOR DEALING WITH CRAVINGS
OUT OF SIGHT, OUT OF MIND

This is more a prevention technique than a coping strategy. You're much more likely to want a drink if it's right in front of you. It's like sweeties at the checkout. If it's right in front of you, calling your name, it's much harder to ignore. So tear up that application for a Saturday job at Oddbins before it's too late.

If you haven't removed all alcohol from the house already, now would be a good time to do so before it starts its siren song and lures you onto (Scotch on) the rocks.

If your partner/flatmate/the voices in your head say it's not fair to ban all booze from the house, consider this: how would they like it if they set themselves a no-TV-for-a-month challenge and you insisted on inviting mates round to watch the latest crime drama every week? Anyway, it's only for one month. Just tell 'em, 'Suck it up, princess,' and at the very least, hide the booze away.

On that note, don't feel the need to test your will power. I mean, if you were on a diet, would you book a tour of Cadbury World? There are temptations enough out there that we don't have control over – in pubs, clubs, supermarkets – so let's just deal with the ones we can control.

CRAVINGS DON'T LAST FOR EVER

The more concentration and energy we give to them – thinking about how much we want a drink, what it's going to taste like, how terrible it is to be suffering a craving – the longer cravings will last.

If the desire for a drink seems to get bigger and stronger and you fear that it won't go away until you give in, here's a brilliant fact: **the average craving lasts for just six minutes.** If you can find a distraction for that time, your craving will diminish.

What could you do in six minutes – make a cuppa, fire off a couple of emails, write a shopping list, phone a friend, craft a funny limerick? Make a list of six-minute fillers so that the next time you get a craving, you've got something else to focus on.

Laura

'When the stress occurs sometimes I think having a drink would be good but the urge so far has passed after a short time.'

CRAVINGS CAN BE SET OFF BY CUES

Cravings can be set off by triggers that set you on the path to wanting a drink. So what's causing your craving? Is it something **internal** like an emotion, a thought, a feeling? Are you bored, stressed, angry, happy? If so, what other pick-me-ups do you use when you're down? How do you celebrate when there's no booze about? Remember the list from Chapter 4 on filling the gap? Remind yourself of these non-alcoholic alternative ways to respond to feelings.

Or is it an **external** cue like the time of day, seeing someone else drinking, the smell of beer, a sunny day? If so, an excellent tactic is to avoid these cues for the next hour or so, if you can. If your craving is still there, niggling, 20 minutes later, chances are you're still in the presence of the trigger that set it off in the first place. Work out what that might be and then move away – physically or metaphorically. If it's a sunny day, grab a good book (preferably this one) and a delicious soft drink and enjoy the sunshine!

If you can't avoid the cue, use some of the other tips overleaf.

Stu

'The first five to seven days were difficult. Drinking had become part of my daily routine. The danger period for me was normally between 7.30 and 9 p.m. – too early to go to bed and too late to call a friend and say, "Hey what are you doing?" So I started to go swimming late in the evening. If I'm going swimming at 9 p.m. of course I can't drink before I go, and I'm not going to open a beer at 10 p.m.'

URGE SURFING

Urge surfing is a sort of mindfulness exercise. Think of the craving as a wave: it starts slowly then builds in intensity to a crescendo before falling away quickly.

If you fight the urge it'll fight back. The more you tell yourself, 'I can't take this craving anymore; I have to do something about it; it's not going away; aaarrgh!' the harder it is to ignore and the longer it sticks around.

So when you feel the desire for a drink, don't fight it. Think about the feeling, rather than the desire for a drink. Sit quietly and focus on how it feels, literally, in your body. What do you notice about the feeling? Keep bringing your awareness back to your senses – how each part of your body feels – and your breathing. Notice when the feelings increase and when they subside – and in a few minutes the urge should start to drain away. Make sure to note down how intense the craving was and how long it lasted in your cravings log at the end of this chapter.

FOOL YOUR BRAIN

As any good magician knows, a little sleight of hand can lead the brain away from what's going on right in front of your eyes. **Your subconscious is totally gullible.** You can tell it anything and it'll believe you. You can fool it into thinking you're having a drink by putting sparkling grape juice in a wine glass or chugging an alcohol-free beer.

The psychology department at South Bank University set up a fake pub on campus to observe students' drinking habits and their behaviour once they'd had a few drinks. The thing is, they weren't necessarily getting what they'd ordered, and the researchers found that placebos work just as well for getting people 'drunk' as the real thing. Cool, huh?

There are some excellent alcohol-free beers on the market, which go great with a curry. There are alcohol-free wines too, plus 'gin and tonic' and other 'spirits' if that's your thing. Some people shy away from alcohol substitutes, but for others it helps with the craving. It's not cheating, it's creative. Take a peek at Chapter 9 for some no-booze drink ideas.

MAKE A SWITCH

Pick something else that you're going to have or do when you get a craving. It has to be something fun or interesting though; completing your tax returns won't help one bit. At least, it doesn't do it for me. Try picking something from your Fill the Gap activity in Chapter 4.

The idea is to break the connection between the craving and the drink by replacing it with something else. If you can always respond to a craving with, say, a chai latte, you'll start to associate the craving with that new thing and not the booze.

GET PHYSICAL

Getting active can help a lot. Even just getting up for a walk around helps channel your energy and can be a good distraction. If you want to take it further, mow the lawn, go for a run or consult Chapter 8. Exercise releases endorphins that can lift our mood so it's a good weapon to have in your craving-busting arsenal. Altering your physical sensations, such as by elevating your heart rate, can dislodge the little craving pest and dissipate its energy.

ANYONE FOR TETRIS?

If not exercise, how about a computer game? You can definitely get your heart rate going and your attention focused elsewhere with a quick jaunt into virtual reality.

Researchers at Plymouth University's Cognition Institute found that playing Tetris helps with cravings. A lot. I kid you not – Tetris! It's something about drawing your whole attention away so that you're absorbed in the game with no space to think about the booze.

Not a Tetris fan? Pick another absorbing distraction. A game of Sudoku, a crossword – anything to hold your attention until the craving passes.

KILL THE ROMANCE

I assume that your relationship with booze hasn't always been wholeheartedly fantastic. Otherwise, why are you here? It's easy to fantasise about how great it would be to have a drink, but try thinking about the last time you drank too much. Recall your last killer hangover; the furry, foul-smelling mouth, the pounding head, the beer sweats. Nice. Remind yourself why having a drink is an unattractive option to stop the urge in its tracks.

Now think about how you'd feel *after* you have a drink – disappointed? Like you've let yourself down? No one likes to feel that way. Focus on how great you'll feel if you don't have a drink. Hopefully that'll compare favourably with the short-lived joy of giving in to the craving monster.

Try reminding yourself of why you want to complete this challenge. Assuming that hasn't changed, you're much closer to achieving it with every day that passes.

And two super simple tips to finish off . . .

- Carry some extra-strong mints. If you feel a craving coming on, pop one in your mouth. Believe me, nothing tastes great after a mint and just the action of sucking that fiery little fella down to a nub can take your mind off it.

- Maybe you're just thirsty. Your brain can interpret this as a desire for a 'drink' drink, not just a drink. When a craving hits, a big glass of water could be all you need!

Sam

'Another technique is that I got really busy in the early morning and late at night. What did I do with all that extra time? Well, I became even more productive!'

→ CRAVINGS LOG

Where was I?	
What was I doing?	
Who was I with?	
How did I feel?	
How intense was the feeling? Rate it out of 10	
How long did it last?	

Where was I?	
What was I doing?	
Who was I with?	
How did I feel?	
How intense was the feeling? Rate it out of 10	
How long did it last?	

Where was I?	
What was I doing?	
Who was I with?	
How did I feel?	
How intense was the feeling? Rate it out of 10	
How long did it last?	

A FINAL WORD ON CRAVINGS

Do you want a drink? Do you really want a drink? Do you? Really, really?

Well, have one, then. No one's stopping you.

You decided to do this challenge, **you** wanted to flex your sober muscle – it's not compulsory and the world won't end if you take a sip of something boozy. So if you really want a drink, then make the decision to have one. (Just one, mind, don't push it!) It's **your** decision. It's nobody's fault, it's just a decision. You can't blame it on a bad day, a hard-drinking best mate or three-for-two at the off-licence. Own it and move on.

Have you failed? Nope, you've just had a drink.

Try Dry is about more than a few weeks without a drink; it's about reviewing your whole relationship with alcohol and challenging your preconceptions about how necessary it is for a full and happy life. If you want a drink, go ahead and don't beat yourself up about it. Maybe this is the exception that proves the rule.

If you do feel that having a drink is a setback, take a look at the next chapter to find out what you can do about it. Or go back to Chapter 4 and take a look at the mindfulness exercises – particularly the one about not judging yourself. Now, dust yourself off and we'll say no more about it.

Maria

'When I've felt bored and wanted a few glasses of wine – I've said to myself, "You'll still be bored but drunk too and will wake with a hangover to boot!"'

—

7. SETBACKS

Me, Myself and I have a setback

Me: Oh, look at that, a nice glass of fizz.

Myself: Mmm, we like fizz. We'd like to be drinking that.

I: Don't listen to Myself, stay strong, ask for an orange juice.

Me: 'Orange juice, please.'

I: Well done, Me. Proud of us. Knew we could do it.

Me: Mmm, nice orange juice.

2 hours later

Me: Oh, look at that, a lovely glass of fizz.

Myself: It'd be great to be drinking that now.

Me: Yes. Yes, it would. After all, I was soooo good earlier, I deserve this.

Myself: Atta girl.

Me: 'Prosecco, please.'

I: Hey! What? Where did that come from? Wait! Stop! Noooooooo!

Me: 'Hic!'

Had a slip-up? Well, that can happen.

Sometimes you can see it happening, almost in slow motion. One half of your brain is already regretting your decision to have a drink and the other half doesn't care.

At other times it just blindsides you. It's a perfectly ordinary day and suddenly there's a half-empty glass in your hand. And not in the metaphorical sense.

These setbacks happen from time to time so we might as well learn from them. In this chapter we take a look at the most common reasons for lapses, so we can understand them, learn from them, and ultimately conquer them!

CYCLE OF (CAKE) CHANGE, OR 'WHY SETBACKS CAN BE HELPFUL'

Welcome to one of my favourite things in the whole world, ever. The cycle of change. This groovy little theory, courtesy of Professor James Prochaska and Dr Carlo DiClemente, explains the processes we go through when we make behaviour changes.

In particular, it explains why I eat cake.

I love cake. There. I've said it. Not just 'Cake is OK, some cake is good, occasionally cake is awesome.' More like, 'Cake is even better than the cycle of change, and that's one of my favourite things in the whole world, ever.' I really, really love cake. No cake is bad cake. Stale cake isn't stale cake – it's a custard delivery system. (Paul Hollywood – if you're reading this, call me.)

This is the cycle of change: change is not an event, it's a process, some of which takes place in our subconscious. As such, we don't always know why we're ready or not ready to make a change but the cogs are turning on the inside. For example, have you ever been on a diet? Well, if you have you will have noticed that sometimes you are in the zone, spurning sugar, dissing full-fat dairy and generally enjoying the satisfying crunch of a stick of celery. At other times, you munch creamy pasta dishes with impunity, giving no thought to calorie content and making a grab for the last slice of garlic bread. Alternatively, you're not actually dieting, but you are flirting with MyFitnessPal and lingering to glance at the latest edition of *Weightloss Weekly* in the newsagents. All part of the cycle, my dears.

There are six stages. Let's take a look at them in turn.

1. Pre-contemplation

In this stage we're happy. Yes, siree, nothing to change here. Others may say: 'Wow, did you eat *all* the lemon drizzle. Again?' but we don't read anything into this. We just enjoy the cake. So too with drinking. Obviously.

2. Contemplation

Change thoughts keep creeping round the edges of our consciousness. I've put on weight; I spend more money on M&S melting-middle chocolate bombes than on heating. That sort of thing. We don't actually do anything, but we do start to think that it would be good to make a change.

3. Preparation

Thoughts become plans. We explore what it might be like to do things differently – weighing up the pros and cons and starting to put things in place for when the change happens. In my case, this means not buying Battenberg and declaring to all who will listen that I'm giving up cake for good this time. For others, it's picking a start date or buying a book about quitting drink for four weeks.

4. Action

This is it! At first we're high on motivation and good intentions. I actually throw cake away at this point. Why not? I'm never eating it again. (N.B. On past attempts I have tried eating all cake in the house the night before I give it up for ever. This does not work. You cannot give up cake by eating cake. It sends completely the wrong message to your oh-so-fickle brain.) You may become evangelical at this point. I know I do. Pointing out helpfully how much saturated fat there is in one-sixth of a family-size chocolate fudge extravaganza. Or reciting all the ways in which eating too much cake can ruin your health.

5. Maintenance

Cakelessness becomes routine and familiarity becomes contempt. You've made the change and kept it going for a while but the gloss has worn off. It's not exciting anymore and your attention moves on to pastures new. You either keep up the change for, say, four weeks until your challenge is done (or you're back down to your fighting pre-cake weight) or you move on to stage six . . .

6. Lapse

'Ah, you mean failure,' I hear you say. Absolutely not. This is where you learn. Failure is stepping off the cycle; lapse is finding out what you need to do to improve your results next time and keeping on pedalling.

The cycle of change was originally developed to describe what goes on, psychologically speaking, when people quit smoking. Professor Prochaska and Dr DiClemente found that, on average, we go round the cycle seven times before making a permanent change. So, there you have it: a slip-up is normal, is to be expected and can even be a positive thing.

Don't get me wrong. I'm not saying, 'Hey, have a few drinks, it doesn't matter.' Of course it does, but be realistic – deal with it and move on. You need to *learn* from a lapse. Not just give up the minute you slip.

COMMON SETBACK STYLES
FALSE STARTS

Day 1: you're committed. You've done the planning, chucked out the vino, posted on Facebook that you're going dry, and then an old friend gets in touch out of the blue . . . only in town for one night . . . let's get together . . . just a couple of drinks . . . Well, it'd be rude not to. And anyway, it's only day 1 so you can start again tomorrow.

If this sounds familiar, you're not alone. The road to hell, as they say, is paved with 'I can start again tomorrow's. Here's what you can do.

Life is short – go! Enjoy! Start again tomorrow.

At this moment the short-term gain (out with a mate) probably outweighs the long-term goal (four weeks) for you. And change is *hard*. We are not a species that greets it with open arms and invites it to dinner.

So. The first one's free. **You have now used your get-out-of-jail-free card**. This is a one-time only offer and tomorrow is day 1 for real.

This deal does not apply if you're actually on day 2 or 3 when your friend rings. Why? Because that way lies madness, or at least not actually getting off the ground with this. If you do get that call a few days in, here's a different plan.

Life is short – too short to fall at the first hurdle.

Go and see your friend and stick to your challenge. You should already have a plan in place for evenings out. If not, flick through to Chapter 10 for some tips. After all, there will be other drinking opportunities throughout the month so you might as well start getting used to them.

Fast forward three weeks. Imagine this: it's day 22 and your friend rings – what would you do? By this time, the chances are you'd tell them about your three weeks off booze and how amazing you feel and suggest you go for coffee or dinner or bowling instead.

So how are you going to get to day 22 if you don't get past day 1, do not collect your £200 and do not pass 'Go'?

Now, get back on that wagon and ride off into the sunset.

CONSTANT RESETS

If you've started on a 28-day challenge once a week for the last month and found yourself constantly pressing the 'reset' button after a few days you need to figure out what's going on.

There will always be circumstances, events, problems and joys that we'd like to experience with a drink in our hands, nothing wrong with that. But what about your goal? Check back in with chapters 1 and 2. Are you still ready, willing and able? If not, you need to work on getting your Try Dry mojo back. Yep, more effort is required. It's worth it, honestly, so go back to basics and figure out what's going on.

IT'S EVERYWHERE!

Here's an experiment for you. Pick one of the following activities:

Walk through the town centre

Watch two hours of commercial television

Read a newspaper

Buy a birthday card

Try out your chosen activity and see how many references to alcohol you can find. Lots, huh? From billboards promoting life-enhancing beers, to three-for-two offers in stores, to TV soaps centred around the pub, alcohol is everywhere you look. No wonder you want a drink. Why wouldn't you, when it's in your line of sight all day?

Does your boss ever reward good work with a bottle of fizz? (Are you the boss – is that what you do?)

Ever noticed how the boozy raffle prizes are always the first to be picked?

What was the last event you celebrated without alcohol?

Hmm, you're probably starting to get the message. We live in an alco-centric society. It's everywhere!

When you start to think about your drinking you become aware of a whole world of pushes to drink that you didn't even know were there. It's like entering the Matrix.

Drinking is not only legal and acceptable, it's seen as the right thing – even the only thing – to do. With all of these pushes to drink, staying strong can be really hard, but not impossible. A few tips, then:

- Consciously notice the alcohol messages and think about who they're aimed at and why. Once you're outside the Matrix and start to see the different 'pushes', they're much easier to resist.

- If it seems as though everyone drinks, it's good to be around all the people who don't, and don't miss it. If you haven't got friends joining you as you Try Dry, check out some of the online communities in the resources section at the end of the book.

- Push back. Make a point of asking for alcohol-free alternatives in bars. Ask for the mocktail list or what the waiter thinks would go well with the fish. Stock up on fancy cordials and make your own concoctions.

EMOTIONAL ARMAGEDDON

Sometimes life kicks you in the teeth and you respond by drowning your sorrows. This is the most common reason why people have a drink when they're committed to not doing so.

It doesn't even need to be a big Armageddon, just something that knocks you off balance emotionally. Then comes the overwhelming desire to scribble out the unpleasantness for a while and deal with the emotions later. You *know* that having a drink will make you feel worse in the long run, but that's also part of its appeal – next to drowning comes wallowing. As booze can make the highs higher and the lows lower, if we go into the glass feeling glum, we're not going to come out smiling.

I've said it before and I'll say it again: This. Is. Normal. But it's not inevitable. Drowning your sorrows makes you internalise negative emotions rather than getting them out there. Try screaming instead. (Maybe just shut the windows first.) Cathartic, isn't it?

Ever watched *The Simpsons*? Of course you have, it's on at least five times a day on four different channels. Here's Marge's advice to a sad young Lisa on dealing with her negative emotions. N.B. This is not good advice.

Marge: Now, Lisa, listen to me. This is important. I want you to smile today.

Lisa: But I don't feel like smiling.

Marge: Well, it doesn't matter how you feel inside, you know, it's what shows up on the surface that counts. That's what my mother taught me. Take all your bad feelings and push them down, all the way down, past your knees until you're almost walking on them. And then you'll fit in and you'll be invited to parties and boys will like you and happiness will follow.

Lisa: (Puts on fake smile)

Marge: That's my girl.

Lisa: I feel more popular already.

That's internalising, and no good ever came of it. There's a lot of advice throughout this book for how you can deal with feelings without turning to alcohol for comfort; try the mindfulness exercise on noticing your thoughts in Chapter 4. Being able to identify what you're feeling is a really good start and prepares you for finding positive strategies to deal with the bad stuff.

DEPRIVATION SYNDROME

OK, this isn't an actual syndrome but it describes that feeling that we get when there's something that we want that we don't think we can have. It comes with all sorts of sneaky thoughts about how we've earned it, or life isn't fair, or we can see others enjoying it so we want it too, or, well, WE JUST WANT IT.

Similar to cravings, deprivation syndrome can pop up unexpectedly for no apparent reason, grab you by the short and curlies, and really test your powers of forbearance.

You can tackle this one by doing a pros and cons list. A what-am-I-gaining/what-am-I-giving-up list, like the benefits list in Chapter 1.

Now go and find yourself a treat. Don't think deprived, think alternative pleasures. I can't stress this enough – you won't enjoy your month if you don't find something fabulous to fill the empty booze hole.

PHYSICAL SYMPTOMS

If you get a couple of days in and the thought of having a drink is increasingly pestering your waking thoughts, or you're feeling physical symptoms such as shakes, sweats, nausea or an overwhelming wave of need for a drink then this challenge isn't right for you at this time. You need to go and see someone about this right away; your GP is often the best place to start.

If you want to quit drinking your local alcohol service can help you to do it safely. If you don't want to quit, they can help you with ways you can feel more in control. Either way, don't just sit there. This is a 30-foot-high flashing neon arrow pointing to taking some positive action. Take the hint before the universe smacks you across the face with a frying pan, as my dear old mum used to say.

NONE OF THE ABOVE

If you're not sure why you had or are moving towards having a little lapse, it could be a SID: a Seemingly Irrelevant Decision. In other words, you found yourself in a position where having a drink just happened and there didn't seem to be a reason.

But SIDs can pretty much always be traced back to earlier events. Often the (unconscious) decision to have a drink was made hours or even days before that actual drink. Your brain just didn't bother telling you what was going on. Brains are like that. They're easy to fool but they can also get their own back and fool you in return. I'd like to give another big plug for mindfulness here. It really helps to have a grip on what your brain is up to behind your back.

Take a look at the scenario below. When do you think the decision to have a drink happened?

Mike

'It was Tuesday at 8 p.m. and I was watching the football on my own at home. My wife came in at about 8.30 p.m. and wanted to chat about something. I told her I was busy but she kept on. We were 2–0 down at half-time so I was really keen to see what would happen. She kept interrupting the game and I missed our goal, about three minutes from time. We lost the match 2-1 and then I had a blazing row with her. I went to bed early and we still weren't speaking the next day.

'When she got home from work on Wednesday evening she wanted to discuss yesterday's argument. That was at about 6 p.m. I decided to go out for a bit of fresh air, thinking we needed time to cool off. I was just going for a walk. I was peckish so I popped into the local chippie and had a bag of chips sitting on the bench outside. I was getting a bit wet in the rain so I thought I'd walk the quick way home, past my local.

'I just found myself outside the pub and it looked warm and dry inside so I thought I'd nip in to see if the lads were there. I had no intention of having a drink. I've stuck to pints of lime and soda for three weeks.

'I saw Jim and he offered me a pint but I said no. We had a chat about this and that and he asked if I was going to the football on Saturday. I told him I couldn't and we talked about the match on telly last night. Jim kept on and on about having a drink even though I said I didn't really want one. He was at the bar and I thought, "A quick one won't hurt." I knew I couldn't be out long because I had to get back and sort things out at home.

'Next thing I know, my glass is empty and I'm getting a round in.'

Poor Mike, he didn't know what had hit him. Here's how the whole thing might have gone with 'brain subtitles' turned on.

Mike (with brain subtitles)

'It was Tuesday at 8 p.m. and I was watching the football on my own at home. **(Brain: A drink would be nice, with the footie.)** My wife came in about 8.30 p.m. and wanted to chat about something. I told her I was busy but she kept on. **(Brain: I just want to watch the football, I've had a hard day and I need some down time.)** We were 2-0 down at half-time so I was really keen to see what would happen. She kept interrupting the game and I missed our goal, about three minutes from time. **(Brain: No way! Best minute of the match. This sucks.)** We lost the match 2-1 **(Brain: Not fair, we didn't deserve that.)** and then I had a blazing row with her. **(Brain: All her fault, now I'm wound up. Could really do with a drink to help get me off to sleep.)** I went to bed early and we still weren't speaking the next day.

'When she got home from work on Wednesday evening she wanted to discuss yesterday's argument. **(Brain: Final straw!)** That was at about 6 p.m. I decided to go out for a bit of fresh air, thinking we needed time to cool off. **(Brain: Yes! Let's go and cool beer, I mean cool off.)** I was just going for a walk. I was peckish so I popped into the local chippie **(Brain: Beer goes well with chips. Just saying.)** and had a bag of chips sitting on the bench outside. I was getting a bit wet in the rain so I thought I'd walk the quick way home, past my local. **(Brain: Perfectly reasonable thing to do – it's raining. No court in the land would convict.)**

'I just found myself outside the pub **(Brain: Oh look, the pub, let's go in.)** and it looked warm and dry inside so I thought I'd nip in to see if the lads were there. **(Brain: The lads we normally have a pint with, that is.)** I had no intention of having a drink. **(Brain: Well, I'm having one.)** I've stuck to pints of lime and soda for three weeks **(Brain: So I'm completely blameless for anything that happens from here on in.)**

'I saw Jim and he offered me a pint but I said no. **(Brain: Yes, please. It's only a matter of time so you might as well give in.)** We had a chat about this and that and he asked if

I was going to the football on Saturday. I told him I couldn't and we talked about the match on telly last night. **(Brain: Football = disappointment = anger = want a pint.)** Jim kept on and on about having a drink even though I said I didn't really want one. **(Brain: Good. Ambiguity – he might try to convince me.)** He was at the bar and I thought, "A quick one won't hurt." **(Brain: Result!)** I knew I couldn't be out long because I had to get back and sort things out at home.

'Next thing I know, my glass is empty and I'm getting a round in. **(Brain: Hee hee hee.)**'

That's SIDs for you.

Mike had the triggers of watching and losing the match, coupled with the emotion of an argument. That's where the SIDs started. Then they lay in wait until the following day. Choosing to walk past the pub, going in, a half-hearted refusal – these were all SIDs that together added up to a great big fall off the wagon.

If you've had an unexpected slip-up, try backtracking to what could have set you up in the hours and even days leading up to it. Once you know what happened you're better armed for next time. Which is where identifying your high-risk situations comes in.

Christos

'I lapsed on Saturday. There was a bottle of wine left over from Christmas. It was only a one-day lapse though. Back on track now and weekdays are easy. It's the weekends that get me.'

LEARNING FROM YOUR SETBACK

So now you know about the cycle of change, you know that a lapse can be a useful guide – if you work to make it so. Here are some tips for making sure your lapse is an opportunity, not a failure.

I'd like to introduce you to Gary Rolfe. You've probably never heard of him, but Gary, Emeritus Professor at Swansea University (and his distinguished colleagues), came up with a so-simple-it's-brilliant model for reflecting on events. Here it is:

What?

So what?

Now what?

Brilliant! Pure genius! These three questions represent how you can look at what happened, its relevance, and what you're going to do about it.

I've adapted them for use in these circumstances but you can use these five little words to reflect on any important event. If you've had a setback, these are great questions to ask yourself:

What?

What exactly happened? What led to the slip-up? What did you drink? What were the consequences? Was it an active choice to drink?

If you weighed up the pros and cons and thought, 'Yes, I want this drink, I'm happy with that decision,' good for you! After all, isn't that what this challenge is about – paying more attention to your drinking? Those four weeks give you the clear space to do that, try it on for size and decide what's next. A little lapse doesn't detract from that. But enough now. Back on the wagon.

If you succumbed to a craving or drinking was a spur-of-the-moment reaction to one of life's little bombshells, here's a golden opportunity to think about how you want to proceed.

So what?

What is the relevance of this? What have you learnt? What do you understand about the things that might trip you up in future?

We're back at mindfulness again. Observe how you felt, but don't judge yourself. If you've had a lapse the worst thing you can do is beat yourself up about it. Negative emotional states can lead to more slip-ups, so think like Master Oogway: what's done is done, so it's time to start planning again.

If you're really concerned by having a drink, talk it through with one of your supporters or share your story on a sober forum. Other people can help you get some perspective on what happened and guide you back on to the straight and narrow.

Now what?

What are you going to do now? What will you do differently next time?

→ Can you identify what actions you could take for a different outcome? Trace back your timeline to see if there was a SID involved. Now replay the scenario with different decisions along the way. Is there a different ending? Have a think about that, and then fill in the table on the next page.

High-risk situation	Options
e.g. Party, ex will be there with new partner	Don't go; go with your new partner/your best mate; take lots of sparkling grape juice; practise mindfulness exercises; plan what to say in advance; have an alternative plan for leaving early; have a treat waiting at home.

AT THE END OF THE CHALLENGE

So, it's a month later. Congratulations! You did it! Well done!

If you had a slip-up, are you telling yourself you failed? A tip: don't do this. Instead, ask yourself, 'Do I feel better for my period of not drinking?' and, 'What did I learn about my relationship with alcohol?' Those are the two real questions.

This challenge was never really about giving up the booze for a month, was it? That was what it looked like, on the surface. But underneath it was about taking a fresh look at your relationship with alcohol. Whatever your reasons for Trying Dry in the first place, it was a signal that you thought a change of some kind would be good.

If you didn't have a slip-up, good for you! You know you can do this now. You can whip out 28/30/31 days of sober any time you want to. Bask a bit. Feels good, doesn't it?

Ten days, 30 days, 50 days, 100 days. It doesn't matter, as long as you're getting what you need from the challenge, asking yourself how you feel, and learning. Setbacks are a big part of that process. They let you know where you might trip up and what your cues for drinking are, and that's vital information to have.

Molly

'Dry January has offered me the opportunity to reassess why I drink and implement my own controls over whether I choose to drink or not.'

—

8. LOVE AND SEX

For those of you who read the chapter titles first and flipped straight to this chapter – go back to the beginning! You don't get to read the saucy bits until you've read the first seven chapters.

Alcohol is often used by people in relationships, new and old, as a way of making conversation flow, as a relaxer, and, well, to get it on. One person going dry can add a little extra twist to any relationship, whether it's two days old or you're approaching your golden wedding anniversary. In particular, it can make dating and sex seem a bit scary.

But actually, being dry can improve relationships and sex. This can be one of the most rewarding aspects of your dry month if you give it a chance. As always, the secret is in the preparation and planning.

Let's start at the beginning.

DRY DATING

If you've not done it for a while – or ever, for that matter – sober dating is a skill that takes practice. The more you do it, the easier it becomes.

Back in the Dark Ages, when I first stopped drinking for a while, it was considered something of a novelty. People would point and stare. But these days, sober is the new black and rather than shun you, you're just as likely to encounter 'No way! Me too!' when you let slip your little secret.

WHY DO PEOPLE HIT THE BOOZE ON DATES?

A Glasgow University study concluded that drunk males and females find each other more attractive than when sober.[*] Really? Who'd have thought?

But there's more to it than 'booze gets you in the mood'. A fascinating experiment in the US explored whether just being around alcohol cues, such as words or images of alcohol, caused men to see women as more sexually attractive.[†] And it did. Even though the men weren't actually drinking, they rated women as more attractive. (The study was repeated with men's opinion of how intelligent women look under the influence of alcohol cues and nope, no difference there.)

A Swiss researcher took this one step further and asked volunteers to rate attractiveness when they thought they'd consumed alcohol, even though they hadn't. Alcohol had been rubbed on the rim of the glass so their drinks smelled like booze. As predicted, under the *expectation* but not the *influence* of alcohol, attractiveness ratings increased. So, if you want to find your partner sexier and them to find you hot in return, replace your aftershave/perfume with whiskey.

There you have it. When it comes to sexiness, our expectations of alcohol influence our perceptions. It's all about how we *think* the alcohol will make us feel. After a few dates without booze, you'll have a much more realistic idea of who you find attractive and who just looks better with beer goggles.

(Sorry that so many of these experiments are about heterosexual couples. More and better research, please, scientists!)

---

[*] Jones, B. T., Jones, B. C., Thomas, A. P., Piper, J., 2003, 'Alcohol consumption increases attractiveness ratings of opposite-sex faces: A possible third route to risky sex', *Addiction 98*, 1069–75.

[†] Friedman, R. S. et al., 2005, 'Automatic effects of alcohol cues on sexual attraction', *Addiction 100*, 672–81.

WHY TRY DATING SOBER

Sober and sexy

Despite all the research into booze and attractiveness, you can still be sexy and sober. Sexier, even. You know what's sexy? Eye contact. Listening more than talking. Smiling. Being confident enough to go on a date sober. Flirting subtly. Wearing clothes you feel comfortable in.

Compare and contrast this with blurry, slurry, stumbly, pukey dating. Puking on a date, or actually on your date, is just gross. They may respond graciously but the chances of them wanting to see you again are slipping further away with every carrot chunk that passes your lips.

In vino veritas

Ever said too much too quickly on a date? Was there alcohol involved? Of course there was. Without booze you're more likely to slow the pace and spend more time getting to know the person. Under the influence of alcohol, we can think that we're a lot closer to someone than dinner and a snog really warrants. Here are a few things you are less likely to do on a sober date:

- Talk about your ex

- Cry

- Talk only about yourself

- Talk too loudly

- Talk too loudly about yourself

- Fall over

- Vomit

- Do something that you'll regret later

- Forget your date's name

- Start flirting with someone else

Reading signals right

You know those dates where everything seems perfect and you think your date is into you and then they don't return your calls? You're confused – it all went so well. That happens a lot less when you're sober dating. If they don't call you'll probably know why, because without a drink you'll be better at reading their signals. You'll also be clearer with your own signals, so you're less likely to find that the other person misunderstands what you think of them based on your booze enthusiasm rather than your true feelings.

PLANNING A DATE

If your usual first-date venue is a bar, sitting in a room full of alcohol and not drinking might seem odd at first, so why not try something different? If there's no pressure to drink because there's no booze about, you can just be yourself.

Coffee shops are always a great option. It's a more relaxed atmosphere, you don't need to dress up – what's not to love? Or how about a museum or an art gallery? Dinner is all very well and good but if the date isn't going well it's bad form to cut and run halfway through the main course. A museum date, on the other hand, can be as long or short as you like. It's also a pleasant change not to feel as though you're at an interview, being stared at across a table and then having that unnecessarily tricky shall-we-split-the-bill conversation. (The answer to this is, obviously, yes: yes you should. Am I right or am I right?)

Go for a walk. Honestly! Walking dates are enjoyable *and* easy. You don't have to worry about keeping up the conversation as you stroll along. You don't have to keep staring into each other's eyes and you're certainly not expected to sink a pint while you do it. Tourist dates can be great fun for the walking option. Go sightseeing in your home town. Find a local landmark or park and take a stroll or a guided tour.

If you don't consider a date a date unless a sit-down meal is involved, try a lunch date. As intimate as the full-blown three-course experience but shorter, cheaper and you get to see your date in daylight. If all goes well, you've got the option of adding on the museum/coffee-shop options later in the day. What's more, there's much less of an expectation that you'll both be drinking.

How about a more active date? Mini-golf, bowling, tennis – they all say: 'Hey, I'm fun and fit and quirky.' If you've got a competitive side (but not an over-competitive side!), this may be the option for you. My mum tells tales of cycling for miles with my dad along country lanes when they were 'courting'. She'd have you believe that every weekend was spent pedalling through gently rolling hills in glorious sunshine, stopping for ice cream and feeding ducks on village ponds, before sitting down to a picnic of tinned-salmon sandwiches, home-made Victoria sponge and lashings of ginger beer. They're divorced now, of course, but don't let that put you off.

FIRST DATES

If there's one time that you'd want a drink to loosen you up, chill you out and put a sparkle in your eye, you'd probably bet that this is it.

Here's a total stranger with whom you may not have things in common, but on whom you want to make a good impression and with whom at some point you might like to have sex; yet you're going to be stone-cold sober. Enough to bring you out in cold sweats? Don't panic!

Yes, alcohol might help you to relax, it might make you feel more confident, it can make conversation easier at first. But it will also make you less you. And it will give you a false impression of your date.

Sober dates can be a bit more awkward. You don't know what to say at first. But hey, this is a first date. It's *meant* to be a bit awkward. Alcohol is just a quick fix. Who promised you that life wasn't going to have awkward moments? What's wrong with being a bit uncomfortable? This is real!

You may think you need a drink to give you confidence or to enable you to talk about yourself and impress the person across the table, but think on this: when was the last time you took some Dutch courage to attend a job interview? It's a stressful situation, in front of strangers and you need to perform at your best, but you probably wouldn't dream of sinking a couple of pints beforehand, would you?

If you think you're going to be stuck for conversation, prepare some questions in advance. I'd particularly recommend open-ended questions that invite your date to open up a bit, like 'Tell me about your work,' rather than 'Where do you work?'

Say something, stupid!

If you get a little tongue-tied around new people without a drink in your hand, why not tell them? This is the case for most of us so why not just get it out into the open and say that you're a little shy until you get to know someone. This is much more attractive than the other option . . .

Say something stupid?

. . . You have one too many and blurt out your entire life story, finishing with a sob at the death of your bunny, Robert Buniro, when you were 15.

SECOND DATES

Once you've got the first date out of the way the second one will probably be easier, but you still have to decide whether you're going to mention the not-drinking thing. There's no reason why you should have to, of course. If you're keeping the dates away from the pub/restaurant/wine-tasting club the question might not even crop up.

How do you feel about your date drinking if you're not? If you're fine being around people who are drinking during your challenge and you're confident you're not going to crumble because you're nervous, second and subsequent dates based on the dinner-and-drinks theme are easier to handle.

If you do find yourself in, say, a wine bar, your date might question your choice of soda and lime. This is what your elevator pitch was made for. Say it and move on. Smile and let them know that you have no problem with them drinking. On the other hand, your date might not feel comfortable drinking whilst you're on the blackcurrant squash, so it's good to iron this one out early on.

That said, you might not fancy being around people drinking, and that's fine too. Drinking is not a great spectator sport so if you are going to find it a struggle to watch your date down a few drinks, continue to avoid pubs and bars for the time being.

When I first took up the challenge, I felt the need to justify not drinking by regaling all and sundry with tales of my drinking shenanigans from times past so that they wouldn't think I was judging them. Take my advice – just don't. No one is impressed by your drinking tales. *Especially* when you're not drinking.

How about if they try to persuade you to drink, or worse, get you a drink after you've said no? This is just rude. Stick to your guns. Take a look at the drink-refusal skills in Chapter 4 for more tips.

ONLINE DATING – TO TELL OR NOT TO TELL

What happens when you put 'not drinking alcohol for a month' in your online profile? You don't have to, of course, but you can if you want to. Why not experiment – see what responses you get with and without a 'no booze' message? If a potential partner thinks it's a big deal and can't get to grips with the idea of going out on a date without a drink you might be better off letting that fish swim on.

The author Catherine Gray reckons it's a good idea to let your potential date know right from the start, and that this might even be attractive to Mr/Ms Right. She discovered research that found online dating profile pictures showing someone drinking are a turn-off and are less likely to get a response than those with no drink in sight. In her words – 'The swipes have spoken!'

RELATIONSHIPS
TWO'S COMPANY

Isaac

'My partner and I are doing Dry January and the results are astounding! We've both lost weight, sleep better, can focus at work, and have better skin. We've been juicing, bathing, gymming more. Just finding more useful things to do than drinking! He says we are reborn!'

If you're in a long-term relationship, or even a new one that you hope will go the distance, you might want to ask your partner if they will join you on your dry sojourn. Not only is it easier to reach your goal for the whole month if you've got a buddy joining in, but you can enjoy the challenge together too.

You won't always find that your partner is as keen for you to go dry as you hope. It might feel quite threatening for them to consider the implications for their own drinking, or they may feel inconvenienced by this change to routine. Stick to your guns and re-read Chapter 3 if you find they're being less than helpful.

If you would like your nearest and dearest to give dry a go, what better way than showing them this book?

Take a minute to think about the main reason for getting your partner to go dry with you:

1. You would like the extra support

2. It will be more enjoyable if you do it together

3. You don't think you can go it alone

4. You're concerned about their drinking

5. You miss doing things together sober

If you chose number four, it's important that you tell them how you feel. However, and this is important: if you use this challenge as a way of trying to change someone else's drinking, you're going to fail. Only they can decide when they want to stop. If you talk openly and honestly about your concerns, they may decide to give it a go. They may not, and that's OK too. This is YOUR challenge, you should be doing it for you. Their challenge will be something they do for them, if and when the time comes.

If your partner does agree to go dry you need to let them take responsibility for that decision. Many's the time I've started a diet and invited poor long-suffering Mr B to join me. Sure, he says, why not. I then proceed to buy, prepare and serve appropriately calorie-controlled meals, reminding him to drink lots of water and adding vitamin supplements where necessary. Day 1 – perfect nutrition. Day 5 – I come home to find him face down in an extra-large, pepperoni double cheese deep pan. Why? Because I didn't give him the opportunity to engage and commit. He wasn't ready, willing and able. He did no planning, no goal-setting – nothing to aim for, no foul if he fails. That's my fault, not his.

If you're getting stuck in and your partner is just leaving it all to you, maybe that's because they didn't want to join you but they don't want to upset you, especially if they agree that it's a good idea in principle, they just don't want to do it. If this is the case, you're going to have to go it alone, with their support, hopefully.

Watching you succeed, seeing how much brighter and happier you are after a month off the sauce, is much more likely to give them the motivation they need to give dry a try.

Drew

'One thing my wife and I did agree was that just because I wasn't drinking it didn't mean that she wasn't drinking . . . I had to square off in my head that if my wife's going to have a glass of wine or whatever there's no point being silly about it. I was doing something that was better for me.'

GOING IT ALONE

Even if you're not inviting your partner to join you for the month, it's a good idea to give them plenty of notice. Just randomly pouring all their favourite wine down the sink one day and declaring your home a dry environment can lead to marital unrest to say the least. Let them know your reasons and your start and initial end dates, then ask for their support.

If you're going to find it difficult to go to the pub/party/wine tasting with them, they'll need a week or two to make other plans. If you need them to not offer you a drink or even not to drink around you, you'll need to discuss this with them in advance. Be kind: this is your choice, but it's not necessarily theirs.

How do you go it alone? This isn't a reason not to go ahead, you just need to plan around it. Here are a few tips to get you started.

Do they have regular drinking habits? If so, it's easy to plan other things to do while they're drinking. If not, ask what they've got planned for the month and choose your alternatives. For example, you may not want to hang out at a concert where there will be lots of drinking but you might be happy to give them a lift, leaving you with a free evening to spend with friends or catching up with that box set in your PJs.

If they're likely to be out carousing into the wee hours, make sure you've got something fun planned so you're not waiting up and counting the minutes.

If not dry, are they prepared to be drier? You might be able to negotiate some new drinking guidelines for the month. E.g. no booze in the house but it's fine when out with friends.

You may be a bit pissed off for the first few days so use your mindfulness practices to notice when you're being miserable and try not to take it out on them.

Let them know your high-risk trigger situations. If you know what might set off a craving it's great to know that you can make the 'get me out of here' face and rely on their support to drop everything and distract you until you feel more in control.

Ask what's different. Sometimes it's our loved ones who notice the benefits of us not drinking for a while. If you're expecting a noticeable weight loss or the energy of a Labrador puppy and you're not getting the result you'd hoped for, those who know you best will be able to point to more subtle changes and that will give your motivation a boost.

Don't mix your messages. Moaning that you can't have a drink will send many loving spouses off to the corner shop to cheer you up with a surprise six-pack. If you have one of these thoughtful partners (they're a keeper!) you can't blame them if you find yourself opening the ring-pull on beer number four two hours later. Check out the information on SIDs in Chapter 7.

Be prepared to fight your corner. On the other hand, your spouse may not agree with your goal and head to the nearest booze emporium in search of sabotage material. Talk to them about why this isn't helpful.

DECODING YOUR LOVED ONE DURING YOUR DRY MONTH

Your partner may be delighted by your Try Dry challenge. They may assume that, as you're not drinking, you'll be happy to drive them around town, listen to their oft-repeated drunken anecdotes, stay up late and then drive them home again whilst they snore loudly in the passenger seat.

But it would be rude to be so obvious about it, so they may develop a more subtle language that, with practice, you should be able to unravel. Here are a few choice phrases that I've picked up from Mr B.

Phrase: 'Are you planning on drinking tonight?'

Of course not.

Translation: 'Would you please drive tonight, o light of my life, so that I can sip of the vine until I am merry?'

Phrase: 'What are you doing on Friday night?'

This sounds promising. Do they have a date in mind? Dinner? Dinner and a show? Don't get your hopes up. If it's your birthday and you've been hinting for weeks, then maybe. But more likely this means:

'There's an acoustic night at the Feathers – any chance of a lift so I can have a pint after? And can you pick me up around 1 a.m.? There's going to be a lock-in.'

Phrase: 'I love you. I really, bloody love you.'

This is tricky. There are two possible translations:

1. 'Look at me, I'm so desirable after three pints, slightly blurry, smelling of curry and swaying, semi-naked in the bedroom doorway at 3 a.m. Want some of this?'

2. 'I'm about to throw up on the bathroom floor. It'd be great if you could clean it up before I go in there with a hangover tomorrow at about noon.'

Phrase: 'You look tired, love. Why don't you get an early night? I'll be up soon.'

Don't fall for this one. Seems innocuous enough but what it really means is:

'Now you're sleeping so soundly, I can stay up playing Xbox/ watching *Love Island* until dawn. Rogue squadrons/evil aliens/ bikini-clad 20-somethings await!'

SOBER SEX

And here's the reason you came to this chapter.

Does not drinking mean you'll get less sex?

Well, maybe, maybe not. But this is definitely an area where that old maxim 'It's quality, not quantity that counts' comes into its own. Just as real sex isn't like porn sex, sober sex isn't like alcohol-fuelled sex.

Drunk sex is easy but sober sex takes a little more thought, a little more patience and a little more time. The effort is worth it. You can really appreciate the emotions and sensations when you're not being battered between the ears by a chemical barrage of arousing hormones. It's just you and your partner. Or partners. Whatever floats your boat.

Now, that can be a scary thought, especially if you generally count on being under the influence to get in the mood. But if you think you *need* alcohol to have sex . . . do I really need to finish that sentence?

Maybe you need to be braver. Maybe you get a little less action, but it will be genuine desire that gets you into bed.

The trick here is to be prepared for a big build-up. Alcohol is known for its aphrodisiac properties so it will get you from 0 to 60 before you can say 'Lamborghini'. It takes time to build desire naturally. It's like the comparison between watching an action film and reading the book. Sure, the film is non-stop car chases and witty one-liners, but with the book you get to explore the characters more, find out their motivation and create your own interpretation.

Sober sex is also likely to lead to better sex long term. You have the headspace to listen to your body. You'll have a better memory of the experience, and so can learn and, more importantly, *remember* what works and doesn't work for you and your sexual partner.

On a purely practical level, having a bit more co-ordination in the bedroom can only be a good thing. Trust me.

Now go out there and have some fantastic sober sex.

Bobbie

'I was drinking a bottle of wine a day. I couldn't wait to settle down with a drink. I looked forward to it all day. I used the Dry January app and soon realised I was addicted to my habits, not to the wine. I haven't touched a drop all month . . . I'm using my gym membership again, I'm also using my evenings much more productively. I feel like a whole person again.'

—

9. STAYING IN

Do you enjoy a drink or two at the end of a hard day to help you unwind? Do you find that nowadays the thought of relaxing in the evening without finishing at least a bottle seems impossible? Welcome to the beer/wine o'clock club.

If you like to drink at home, it's so easy to rack up the units without even thinking. It's right there in the fridge – how convenient! No need to drive, no need to make an effort to interact with anyone, you can just sit and chill. You don't even need to get drunk – just a few glasses to take the edge off, and boy does it take the edge off. Except when it encourages you to wallow in just how rotten the day was.

If you're on your own, there's no one to complain that you're hogging the booze, and if you're with friends, well, it's hard to tell who's had what, and you're all in the same boat, so why not?

What on earth do you *do* in a dry month of evenings at home, then?

You do other things, that's what. Fun things; things you've been meaning to get round to; new things; relaxing things. Now that you've got some extra free time, you can start to explore ways to spend it. If you're usually too tired to do any kind of exploring by the end of the working day, you'll be surprised at how much more energy you have once your sleep patterns improve and you're not still a wee bit hung-over from the night before.

In Chapter 10 I've given you a whole list of fun things you can do during your dry month – but many of them involve Leaving The House. If you just want a night (or a day) in without booze, here are seven things to try.

SEVEN NIGHTS IN HEAVEN (OR AT LEAST IN YOUR HOUSE)

1. Listen to music

Get out your old vinyl, dust off your mix tapes, polish your CDs, fire up Spotify, sit back and just listen. Music is so often the backing track to our lives that we don't think to stop and make it the main event. Why not spend an evening putting a playlist together? It might be a collection of calming tunes, or an evening of nostalgia with the soundtrack from your life. Either way, listening to music is a great way to relax.

2. . . . Or make music yourself!

If you already play an instrument, you could spend an evening getting back into practice. An hour or two a couple of times a week will soon have you strumming, drumming, blowing or tinkling the ivories like a rock star. If you don't already play but have always wanted to, you can pick up a bargain instrument on eBay, watch a few 'how to' YouTube videos and off you go. After all, that's how Justin Bieber got started.

3. Garden glory

This is one of those things that you either love or hate. If you're a passionate gardener, you're probably out there already on a regular basis. If not, I'm not suggesting you get all Monty Don; just plant a few bulbs in a window box or sprinkle some herb seeds in containers. If you don't have the space or a garden of your own, why not get involved in a community garden near you? Remember to water your seedlings regularly – they do moist, not dry – and by the time your dry month is over, you should see your plants starting to grow. Symbolic, isn't it?

4. Pamper yourself

Why not treat yourself to the whole shebang? Give yourself a manicure, a pedicure, face-mask and a mineral soak in the bath. Stick an intensive moisture treatment on your hair and let your worries drift away. You could invite a friend over for mutual pampering and a chat whilst you sip herbal 'detox' tea. Believe me, blokes, this is for you too.

5. Get creative

Maybe you can knit, maybe you like to whittle, maybe you've never tried either but would like to give it a go. You don't have to be brilliant at it, you just have to enjoy the process. There's something deeply satisfying about creating something from scratch, and I don't mean a vodka martini. Try out different creative arts to see what you enjoy.

Don't fancy something creative, but do like the idea of learning? Check out the wide range of (free) courses available online.

6. Plan a holiday

Long gone are the days of just picking up a brochure, choosing a hotel and leaving the rest to the package-holiday touts. These days it's all about creating your own bespoke experience. The plethora of holiday websites can take a bit of wading through so why not commit an evening to planning the perfect getaway? It doesn't have to be a long-haul extravaganza (beware the 'all-inclusive' option), just getting excited about a weekend away is a fun way to pass the time.

7. Spring cleaning

OK, not everyone will find this relaxing but it can certainly be cathartic and rewarding. If you've got a cupboard, loft or room that could really do with a sort-out, it's a useful way to spend an evening. Not only are you creating extra space, you can donate anything you don't want to charity for that feel-good factor or raise a bit of cash selling it online. Time passes quickly once you start delving into your hoard of forgotten items and you won't even think about drinking once you're up to your eyeballs in old lampshades, bicycle chains and inflatable dolphins.

Gwen

'We haven't missed the pub and if anything have found other things to do.'

—

WHAT TO DRINK WHEN YOU'RE 'NOT DRINKING'

Whatever you miss about alcoholic drinks (except the alcohol), there's a drink option to fill the gap in this handy guide.

🍹 MOCKTAILS

All the fun, none of the hangover! Here are some of our favourite mocktail recipes. Try out a couple for a good night in.

—

PEACH ICED TEA

This is a refreshing, sophisticated cooler for summer evenings.

Ingredients	Method
275ml peach iced tea slice of lemon slice of orange sprig of sage ice cubes	Place slices of lemon and orange along the rim of a tall glass, facing outwards. Fill the glass with ice and iced tea, finishing off with the sprig of sage and a paper straw.

—

CHERRY EXPLOSION

An exciting party mocktail with lots of flavour and a bit of fizz.

Ingredients	Method
10ml grenadine syrup 25ml cherry syrup 160ml lemonade wedge of lime ice cubes	Fill a highball glass three quarters full of ice. Shake the syrups together and pour into the glass. Top with the lemonade and stir. Garnish with the lime wedge.

SPICED APPLE

This is an autumn favourite!

Ingredients

275ml apple juice
50ml cola
shake of cinnamon
wedge of lemon
slice of apple

Method

Fill a highball glass with ice.
Pour in the apple juice then
top up with cola. Sprinkle with
cinnamon to taste and garnish
with lemon and apple.

—

MULLED APPLE

The perfect winter warmer.

Ingredients

1.5l apple juice
2 cinnamon sticks
 (plus more for decoration)
6 whole cloves
½ tsp allspice
1 orange, cut into slices
1 lemon, cut into slices
50ml maple syrup

Method

Pour the apple juice and maple
syrup into a large pan. Add the
cinnamon, cloves and allspice
and heat gently until not quite
boiling. Add most of the orange
and lemon slices and simmer
gently for one minute. Strain
into cups or mugs and garnish
each with a fresh cinnamon
stick and a couple of slices of
the fruit.

Deb

**'Sparkling water, basil and cucumber slices,
that's very refreshing. Tonic and lime.
I started getting creative with different
mocktails. My friend and I discovered that
they're just as good – better!'**

SQUASH SUPREME

A fantastic thirst-quencher, very fruity and great for any occasion.

Ingredients

100ml pink grapefruit squash
 (made up with water)
100ml lemon squash
 (made up with water)
50ml orange juice
50ml soda water
slice of grapefruit
slice of lemon
ice cubes

Method

Half fill a tall glass with ice.
Pour in the squash and orange
juice. Top up with soda and
add grapefruit and lemon
slices.

—

TROPICAL SUNRISE

As the days of spring start to lengthen into summer, this is a
great drink for those first warm evenings of the year.

Ingredients

150ml mango juice
150ml fiery ginger beer
15ml lime juice
10ml grenadine syrup
ice cubes

Method

Half fill a glass with ice cubes
then top with the juices and
ginger beer. Pour the syrup
slowly down the inside of the
glass to create a sunrise effect
of red at the bottom and
orange on top.

🥷 CLASSICS REINVENTED

Here are a few of my favourite cocktails, just without the booze.

—

SINLESS SANGRIA

Not only a great al fresco drink, but one of your five-a-day too.

Ingredients

450ml boiling water
2 teabags
2 cinnamon sticks
100g caster sugar
450ml pomegranate juice
150ml orange juice
 (fresh if possible)
3+ fruits of your choice cut into
 thin slices, e.g. orange, lemon,
 apple, grapes, strawberry, lime
450ml soda water
ice cubes

Method

Pour the boiling water over the teabags and cinnamon sticks and steep for 3–4 minutes. Discard teabags and stir in sugar until dissolved. In a large pitcher combine the tea, cinnamon, juices and fruit. Refrigerate for at least one hour so that the fruit soaks up the liquid. Add the soda and ice cubes just before serving.

—

NO-JITO

An old favourite – make sure you give the mint leaves a good pounding.

Ingredients

handful of mint leaves
50ml fresh lime juice
1 tbsp agave syrup (or honey)
200ml sparkling water
crushed ice
wedge of lime

Method

Tip the mint leaves into a tall glass and muddle to release the oils. Top the glass up with the crushed ice. Add the lime juice, water and syrup and stir until dissolved. Garnish with extra mint leaves and lime.

MOCK-A-RITA

Based on the margarita, this is an elegant and not-too-sweet drink.

Ingredients

200ml coconut water
50ml lime juice
1 tbsp agave syrup (or honey)
juice of half an orange
lime and salt for glass rim
strip of orange zest
crushed ice

Method

Shake some salt onto a small plate. Squeeze lime round the rim of a margarita glass and then dip into the salt. Mix the other ingredients in a cocktail shaker and strain into the glass. Garnish with orange zest.

—

MOCK-A-POLITAN

A classy cocktail-hour drink, and rather moreish.

Ingredients

50ml cranberry juice
200ml coconut water
25ml lime juice
1 tbsp agave syrup (or honey)
crushed ice
strip of lime zest

Method

Pour ingredients into a cocktail shaker then strain into a cosmopolitan glass. Garnish with lime zest.

—

MOSC-NO MULE

All the kick but none of the booze.

Ingredients

150ml fiery ginger beer
50ml soda water
3 tbsp fresh lime juice
crushed ice
wedge of lime

Method

Fill a tumbler three-quarters full of crushed ice. Top up with ginger, soda and lime. Stir and garnish with lime.

👁 OTHER ALCOHOL-FREE ALTERNATIVES

Mocktails not your thing? There are still plenty of delicious alcohol-free alternatives for you to try. Even your local supermarket is likely to stock more than one brand of alcohol-free beer, wine and even a spirit or two, not to mention non-alcoholic fruit ciders and an exotic range of cordials.

The following drinks all get the thumbs-up from our hardworking taste testers. It's a tough job but someone's got to do it.

Alcohol-free or low-alcohol?

In the UK, drinks that contain 0.05 per cent alcohol (ABV) or less are considered alcohol-free, whilst drinks of up to 1.2 per cent are considered low-alcohol. Here our taste testers have included wines, ciders, spirits and beers of up to 0.5 per cent ABV. We don't consider 0.5 per cent ABV drinks 'cheating' during a dry month – but it's up to you to make your own rules!

Wines

You can turn up to a house party with a bottle of one of these and nobody will be any the wiser. Fill your wine glass to the brim and tuck in to the cheesy nibbles at will.

Reds

Rawson's Retreat Cabernet Sauvignon ABV 0.5 per cent

Without doubt, this is one of the best low-alcohol reds. And to be honest, we've tasted plenty of normal-strength red wines that don't come close to this quality. It actually tastes like a Cabernet Sauvignon and has a good, deep red colour. Whatever it is they do to take the alcohol out of a wine without removing the pleasure, Rawson's Retreat do it well. The bottle design, with an image of the vineyard, gives it the look of a proper wine; not just some alcohol-free stuff you have to put up with. Its major advantage over many of the wines out there on the market is that it isn't loaded with sugar, and is delightfully low in calories.

Torres Natureo Syrah ABV 0.5 per cent

Making a decent low-alcohol red is tricky. According to Miguel Torres Maczassek, the secret of this wine is the technological wizardry of the Spinning Cone Column, which removes the alcohol without destroying the flavour. He may be right. It looks like wine, smells like wine, and tastes almost like wine. Overall, it's got a good colour and nice blackberry taste. We found it went down well with a spaghetti bolognaise.

Whites

Rawson's Retreat Semillon Chardonnay ABV 0.5 per cent

Amongst the low-alcohol white wines, this Australian number stands out. It's got the yellow tinge of a well-oaked Semillon Chardonnay. It smells like Chardonnay, and it's not sugary at all. There's a little bit of a sour aftertaste, but on the whole, if you love white wine and you're looking to lay off the booze, this is probably your best shot.

Like all the Rawson's Retreat wines, it's well presented in a bottle that makes it look like a decent wine. Good enough to fool your friends if they're not privy to your Try Dry challenge.

Rosé

Tesco Ganarcha Rosé ABV 0.5 per cent

This rosé is the work of the well-established Spanish wine makers Felix Solis. They've been turning grapes into vino for more than 30 years and make a lot of wines you've probably heard of. We thought this one had a really good full fruity flavour. As you might expect for a rosé, it's a bit sweet, but not overly so. On a very practical level, our taste testers emptied the bottle pretty quickly, so something about it was enticing us to keep topping up! Low-alcohol wines don't get much better than this.

Torres Natureo Rosado ABV 0.5 per cent

Torres Natureo Rosado was launched in 2013, along with the red. We thought this one smelt of strawberries, which is always a good start! It's got a good rosé colour too. If anything, it's actually a bit too dry for a rosé, but that's no bad thing amongst its overly sweet competitors.

Sparkling

Rawson's Retreat Chardonnay Pinot Noir Muscat
ABV 0.5 per cent

Sparkling wines mean celebrations. So wouldn't it be great if joining in the festivities didn't mean the non-drinkers raising a glass of orange juice while everybody else has champagne? This wine may be the answer. It's nicely packaged, with a proper cork, and looks like something you'd buy for a special occasion.

Once poured, it's got a great colour and plenty of bubbles. No, it's not the best sparkling white in the world, but we've had much worse full-strength fizz at weddings and christenings over the years. The days of raising a glass of orange juice to the happy couple may be at an end.

Sainsbury's Sparkling Wine ABV 0.5 per cent

This one pours well with plenty of bubbles and it keeps its fizz. The colour's a little pale, but taste-wise it's nice. There's a little bit of sweetness but not too much, with a certain Champagne-like sharpness. Like the Rawson's Retreat sparkling wine, this one comes in a nice dark green bottle and has a proper cork, which just makes it feel a bit more special.

Beers

More and more pubs and restaurants are sticking one or more alcohol-free beer options on their menu, and about time too. Here's a selection of beers to suit all tastes.

Drew

'I rediscovered ginger beer, squashes – the drinks that you'd expect. But the revelation for me was low-alcohol and no-alcohol beer, which I'd previously pooh-poohed. Because some of my friends were doing Dry January as well, we all had our own ideas about the best ones. A friend had been to Germany for a week and he came back with a view on the German low-alcohol beer market. They have it on tap over there apparently!'

Lagers

Jupiler 0.0 ABV 0.0 per cent

Jupiler is very big in its home country of Belgium. So, can the 0.0 per cent version match that success? We'd have to say yes. It's a really good lager. It's got the right colour, the right aroma, and a nice rounded flavour with just a hint of herbs. If lager's your thing, you won't be disappointed.

Cobra Zero ABV 0.0 per cent

If you've ever had a curry, you've probably had a Cobra. The aim with this beer was to brew a beverage that was less gassy than most lagers and less bitter than traditional ales, especially for drinking with Indian food. Taste-wise, we'd say that Cobra Zero has a smooth flavour and is surprisingly malty for a lager. It goes well with Indian food, of course, but shouldn't be kept just for curries, as it makes a decent accompaniment to any dish. The presentation of this beer is great, using a green glass version of the iconic Cobra bottle (elephants, crossed swords and all).

Cobra Zero also guarantees itself a diverse audience by being approved by the Vegetarian Society and certified kosher by the London Beth Din.

Heineken 0.0 ABV 0.0 per cent

When Heineken launched their first ever alcohol-free beer in March 2017, with a £2.5 million marketing campaign, it was a sure sign that the 'dry' drinks market is one the big players are taking seriously. Heineken are making a big push to get their new beer out to pubs and bars. Like Carlsberg 0.0, it comes in a smart bottle that cries out, 'Drink me while you're watching the footie on the big screen!' Like Erdinger, Heineken are also hoping to attract health-conscious consumers, and the bottle has some very comprehensive nutrition information on the back. It looks, smells and tastes like a great lager. It pours well, with a nice colour and a decent head, and it has none of the unpleasant aftertaste that mars so many other zero-alcohol beers.

Becks Blue ABV 0.05 per cent

An old favourite. Good with curry, nice with lime. Becks Blue has been around for so long it's mainstream. Available in cans or bottles, most supermarkets and lots of pubs sell it. It's not too sweet and has a slightly hoppy finish.

Dark Ales

St Peter's Without ABV 0.0 per cent

Although purists may quibble, it could be called the first 'alcohol-free real ale'. It's aimed at drinkers who like to take their time over a drink. As for the beer itself, it knocks most alcohol-free beers out of the ring and it's better than most of the big-brand 3.5 per cent or 4 per cent bitters you'll find in cans or on tap. It's got a lovely nutty colour, pours well with a good head on it, and it's got a great malty flavour.

Golden Ales

St Peter's Without Organic ABV 0.0 per cent

Just when you thought it couldn't get any Withoutier, there's another one – organic this time. And it's approved by the Vegan Society, so it's extra planet-friendly as well as being good for your liver. If you want to protect the environment and avoid a hangover, here's your beer! Appearance-wise, this is a very pale beer, almost like a German weissbier, but taste-wise it's a very British ale.

Leeds Brewery OPA ABV 0.0 per cent

Two years in the making, this traditional English pale ale is just delicious. It's a bit hoppy and pretty malty, but not too much of either. And it looks great too. It's got a lovely caramel colour. The whole brand and bottle design has obviously been well thought out.

Stouts

Nirvana Kosmic Stout ABV 0.0 per cent

Once poured, it's got a beautiful dark chocolate colour. There's a hint of liquorice in the taste, but what it reminds us of most is Lyle's black treacle (a blast from the past that brought back an *Oor Wullie*-related Proustian memory for one of our beer tasters). There's none of the bitterness you'd usually expect in a stout. So, if you're looking for a take on a traditional stout, we'd probably point you in the direction of other alcohol-free stouts. On the other hand, if you fancy trying one of the most original and inventive dark beers on the market, grab yourself a bottle of Kosmic.

Ciders

Kopparberg Alcohol-Free Mixed Fruit
ABV not more than 0.05 per cent

As their makers are the first to admit, Kopparberg ciders are sweet. Very sweet. They don't look much like cider either. If you're a cider connoisseur (or cider snob, depending on how you look at it), you probably won't like them very much.

That said, there clearly is a huge demand for sweet, easy-drinking ciders and if you're part of this growing trend, then this may be just the drink for you.

Kopparberg Alcohol-Free Pear Cider
ABV not more than 0.05 per cent

According to the people at Kopparberg, the juices of plump pears are mixed with naturally soft water to make something fruity with the 'punch of a strong pear taste'.

As with other Kopparberg ciders, this one is never going to get the votes of cider purists, but should go down well with drinkers who've enjoyed the sweeter, easier-drinking ciders that have come onto the market since around 2000. We tried both the Kopparberg full-strength and alcohol-free pear and mixed fruit ciders side-by-side and we couldn't tell them apart.

Spirits

Alcohol-free spirits are the new kids on the block. Not to everyone's taste but, then again, what is? So, if you like a challenge, and you obviously do because you've made it to Chapter 9, then why not give these adventurous little numbers a try?

Seedlip Spirit 94 and Garden 108 ABV 0.0 per cent

These have to be some of the most unusual additions to the alcohol-free drinks world. They're marketed as 'the world's first non-alcoholic spirits'. It may be a matter of how you define that, since drinks claiming to be alcohol-free whiskeys have been around since the 1990s (although not always well received!).

Once we'd bought them, our next question was how to drink them. We tried them neat to start off with. This is obviously not how they're intended to be drunk – the flavours are way too strong for that. They come with serving suggestions – premium tonic for the 94 and elderflower tonic for the 108 – so we had a go at that. The result is two very light, very clean drinks. We could imagine drinking them on a riverboat trip on a summer's evening. This is not G&T. In fact, we're still not sure what it is, but if you're in the market for unexpected flavours, give it a go.

The bottle designs really set these drinks apart as top end. Looking at the nutritional information, they are calorie-free, so the only calories you might want to think about are the ones in your tonic.

Teetotal G'n'T ABV <0.5 per cent

Launched in 2015, this is a very different drink to Seedlip – much more like a conventional gin-based drink. According to the company, during their taste testing with more than 10,000 people, the vast majority of people could not tell that this was a non-alcoholic drink. Neither could we.

There's a good backstory to this drink too, and to the Yorkshire-based company that makes it. A publican, a research chemist and an entrepreneur decided it was time to come up with an adult alternative to fizzy pop for people who weren't drinking. The aim was to produce something as good as its alcoholic equivalent, using only natural ingredients and keeping the sugar content low – a drink that was 'not too sweet, something which made you feel part of the party, but without the alcohol'. They may well have succeeded.

It comes premixed in 200ml bottles, matching the trend for ready-to-drink bottles and cans of spirits and mixers in the major supermarkets.

There's an alcohol-free alternative for every occasion. And if you don't fancy an alcohol substitute, why not check out the wide range of tonics and fruit juices that are available? Iced tea is back in vogue and kombucha is taking the market by storm. (It's a fermented tea drink and apparently it keeps you regular, if you know what I mean. Bonus!)

So there's no reason why your evenings in during your dry month can't be as relaxing and delicious as ever (and the mornings after significantly better). Cheers!

Jess

'I've learnt that alcohol doesn't have to be part of my weekly life, which honestly I didn't think was possible.'

—

10. GOING OUT

If you think that taking a dry month means locking yourself away from the world while your friends carouse nightly 'til the wee small hours, think again. Maybe you don't think you can survive a wild night out on just orange juice, and sure, it can be daunting to imagine how you're going to enjoy hours of socialising without the booze. But there's more to making merry than getting drunk.

The last few years have seen an exponential rise in the number of venues catering for the savvy non-drinking customer. Where once the choice was limited to fruit juice, cola or water (sparkling, if you were feeling a bit risqué), there are now hundreds of great drinks available in pubs, clubs and even wine bars across the UK – though there's still room for improvement.

That's not to say that going out dry is challenge-free. In this chapter I'll talk you through some of the perks and pitfalls.

PLANNING

Yes, you've heard this before, but it's worth repeating. Make your plan for evenings out well in advance. Whether that's about offering to drive to take temptation out of the picture or deciding in advance to cut and run early, the more you anticipate situations that might make you want a drink, the more likely you are to avoid the pitfalls, Wile E. Coyote.

Andrew

'We all went out for dinner at a local pub. There were some big personalities there – I knew the conversation would be quite loud and full on and I walked into the pub thinking, "I'm going to be feeling left out; I'll feel not interesting or engaging to other people." But I had one of the best nights ever. The conversation felt much more alive, I could hear what people were saying, I felt confident. It was weird. It was totally the opposite of what I was expecting.'

SHALL I STAY OR SHALL I GO?

It's wise to choose carefully which invitations you'll say yes to and which you'll give a miss this month. Some occasions might just be a chore, or too much of a challenge, when you're not drinking.

If you get an offer and you're not sure whether to accept or not, say you need to check your diary and give yourself a chance to think it through. It's easy to rush to accept and then, on reflection realise that it's going to be hard to resist a drink – but you don't want to let the host down, so you go and feel miserable (either because you want a drink or because you have a drink). So give yourself some time to weigh up the pros and cons before you reply.

If you really want to go to a boozy event, or one where you know you'll be tempted to drink, it's worth reflecting on whether that desire might be because you are, in your heart of hearts, planning to drink.

Remember: saying no to an event isn't the end of the world. In fact, being able to say no to events you don't want or it wouldn't be wise to go to is a skill that will stand you in good stead long after your dry month is over!

If an event you *have* to go to is likely to be particularly trying and drink-inducing – your ex's wedding or a funeral for example – figure out your coping strategies in advance. Make sure you've got someone to turn to if you become emotional. You need someone who will remind you that having a drink at this point is a bad idea.

WHAT'S YOUR PARTY TIPPLE?

Another important part of your plan is to decide on your drinks for the evening in advance, using the suggestions in Chapter 9 for inspiration. Yes, I know this might seem to take the spontaneity out of things, but if this is your first big evening out, plan, plan, plan. If you go completely off-piste you could end up mixing grapefruit juice and cola, which I've tried, and it's disgusting.

SPECIAL EVENTS

If there's a not-to-be-missed but boozy special occasion – a wedding, a christening, a landmark birthday – here are a few tips:

- Let the host know in advance that you're not drinking to avoid any embarrassment when it comes to the toast.

- If you want to celebrate with a particular drink that will help you feel part of the fun, like one of the fancy non-alcoholic options from Chapter 9, bring it along with you. Prepare to have to share with (or fend off!) other people who'll be eyeing your hangover-free, delicious option!

- Feel a bit smug. You get to have fun at the event and you won't have a sore head or the 'what did I do or say?' panic in the morning; a.k.a. beer fear!

- Many of us associate these big events with alcohol, so it can be hard to imagine attending without drinking. But when you think about it – properly think about it – is the alcohol really what makes a wedding, or a christening, or a big birthday of someone you love special? What about the getting dressed up, the celebration itself, the awkward speeches, the dancing? Try to think about the fabulous bits you still get to enjoy – not the one bit you don't.

DRINK-REFUSAL SKILLS

If you've read Chapter 3 on relationships, you're already skilled up! If you need a refresher it's worth popping back there before your first night out, as being able to refuse drinks calmly and confidently will really help you to enjoy your evening.

EARLY NIGHT

One big difference when you're off the booze is that you may not be able to stay awake until the early hours. That's because alcohol can disrupt our perception of time so the hours fly by. Without the booze-fuelled FOMO you can make a more rational decision as to whether you want to party on or wind things up. It's not boring to be ready for some Zs at midnight. If you've had enough of the party just say your goodbyes and head home for a good night's sleep.

Don't *expect* this to happen though. Booze sends some of us straight to sleep (even if the sleep we get isn't particularly restful). If that's you, you might just find yourself partying the night away as never before during your dry month, rather than being propped up on a pile of coats in the corner.

If you do find it harder to stay out late as you Try Dry, this can be tricky if you go to an event with someone who wants to party on. You'll need to sort this one out before you head off so that you don't sit staring at your watch while your partner/mate dances 'til dawn, or they don't feel let down when you head off before they're ready to flop.

If you do want to stay the distance, there's no shame in having an early-evening nap to keep you going a bit longer. I won't tell – it'll be our secret. Another trick to finding your second wind is to top up with some strong coffee. Beware, though, you have to get the timing right or you'll still be wide awake when everyone else is ready for home.

If you're really not up to going out on the town without a drink there's a whole world of other activities to explore later in the chapter. You could even check out one of the 'dry' bars below.

WHERE TO GO FOR A GOOD BOOZE-FREE NIGHT OUT

These venues or events aren't simply sober-friendly – they're built entirely for people who aren't drinking.

The Brink

15–21 Parr Street, Liverpool L1 4JN

www.thebrinkliverpool.com

Liverpool's original and first dry bar and restaurant. They do an amazing range of mocktails and the vibe is fantastic.

Morning Gloryville

www.morninggloryville.com

Think you can't dance sober? Think again. If you're an early riser, you HAVE to check out MG's morning rave events. Strut your stuff from 6.30 a.m. and enjoy a full-on, alcohol-free party atmosphere. Don't forget to bring your dancing pants. Morning Gloryville have held events in London, Liverpool, Brighton, Leeds, Birmingham and Manchester. Check out their website to find the latest raves.

Redemption Bar

**320 Old Street, London EC1V 9DR
or 6 Chepstow Road, London W2 5BH**

www.redemptionbar.co.uk

A bar. But dry. Classic pub feel and great healthy food menu.

George Street Social

45–51 George Street, Newcastle upon Tyne NE4 7JN

www.roadtorecoverytrust.org.uk

Founded by the Road to Recovery Trust, this is an alcohol-free café run by people in recovery with extras like meeting rooms, workshops, dance classes and more. Great coffee too.

Café Sobar

22–24 Friar Lane, Nottingham NG1 6DQ

www.doubleimpact.org.uk/cafe-sobar

Live music, poetry, DJs, a great atmosphere and no booze. A fab place to mingle and soak up the relaxed vibe. This makes for a chilled change from Nottingham's more rowdy local bars.

Fitzpatrick's Temperance Bar

5 Bank Street, Rawtenstall, Rossendale, Lancashire BB4 6QS

The oldest temperance bar in Britain. Take a trip down memory lane and try the Fitzpatrick range of old favourites including dandelion and burdock, sarsaparilla and blood tonic. More of a shop than an actual bar and well worth a visit if you're in the area.

WHERE TO EAT OUT?

Restaurants are also getting wise to the trend for booze-free drinks. Some of the larger chains offer a range of mocktails and other non-alcoholic options for the discerning Try Dryer, such as Café Rouge, Chiquito and Pizza Hut. It's worth checking out your local independent restaurants too, as many of them will have alcohol-free options. You can find some real hidden gems, and amazing new drink flavours that you'd never have noticed when just skimming the menu to see if they have your 'usual'.

WHAT SHALL I DRINK WITH DINNER?

If you're eating out, it's handy to have some alcohol-free options that are going to enhance your dining experience. If you're at a restaurant you can ask your waiter what would suit your food choice. I've had some blank looks when doing this but also some amazing suggestions, including one venue that invented a lavender-infused mojito-style mocktail, just for me! I tipped well, told all my friends and it became my favourite restaurant.

If you'd rather just go with the flow here are a few 'standard' drinks that complement the flavours of classic meals.

Aperitif

A good tonic water with lemon or lime sharpens the appetite and doesn't look out of place.

Chicken

Chicken will go with pretty much everything, so for a refreshing change try cranberry and raspberry or any fruit juice topped up with lemonade.

Fish

Elderflower pairs well with the delicate flavour of most fish. Choose either a sparkling pressé or mix up a cordial with sparkling water. Robust fish such as salmon or sardines can take something a little more hearty, such as a St Clements mocktail (orange juice and bitter lemon).

Beef

A cloudy apple juice with a twist of lime complements beef dishes perfectly. For a touch of nostalgia, why not try it with dandelion and burdock too.

Lamb

Berry cordials bring out the flavours of this rich meat as long as they're not too sweet. Cherry colas also work well with lamb.

Pork

A classic pairing with pork is ginger, so a ginger ale or apple and ginger cordial will work well. Blackberry cordial is also delicious with pork.

Pasta

For creamy pasta dishes, soda and lime cuts through to refresh the palate, and for tomato-based dishes a light tonic works well.

Seafood

Something lime-based such as the classic lemonade and lime or a lime pressé tone well with the sweetness of mussels, scallops or prawns.

Dessert

This is easy. Fresh coffee is the perfect partner to a tasty dessert.

Cheese

Tomato works with cheese on a pizza and it works here – so try tomato juice with the cheese course. If you like, add a dash of Worcester sauce.

RANDOM ACTIVITY GENERATOR

Don't fancy a night out on the town but stuck for something to do? If you're after adventure rather than relaxation, or want to get out and about rather than stay in, we've come up with an activity for every day of the month. Some require a little more, er, planning than others (number 17, anyone?) but all are guaranteed alcohol-free fun.

All you have to do is pick a number between 1 and 31 and take a look at the list below. Whatever activity corresponds with your chosen number – that's your challenge to complete before the month is out.

1. **Go to your local coffee shop** for a lazy Sunday latte. This is a nice bonus if you don't normally see Sunday mornings as you're usually sleeping off Saturday night until after midday.

2. **Volunteer** your time. Your local volunteer centre will be able to put you in touch with a worthy cause that you can get involved in (you can find your nearest one at navca.org.uk). You can give as little or as much of your time as you feel able. There are lots of types of volunteering, including micro-volunteering (a few minutes here and there) and professional volunteering (where you apply the skills you've developed throughout your career).

3. **Visit a museum.** Local history, natural history or all manner of interesting collections can be found in museums. Seek out one that intrigues you.

4. **Go bowling.** It's retro so it's in!

5. **See a local football/rugby/cricket match.** Go along and cheer on your local team. Grassroots support is always welcome and you'll really get into the spirit of things – just watch out for that post-match celebration.

6. **Learn to knit.** Another retro pastime that's making a come-back, this is one for gals and fellas alike – you won't believe how relaxing it is.

7. **Attend a mocktail-making class.** These are springing up in cities all over the country.

8. **Take a trip to your local nature reserve.** What better way to spend a few hours than in the great outdoors. Check out the National Trust, the RSPB and Natural England websites for local reserves.

9. **See a musical or play.** Your local am dram might be putting on a production – you could even sign up to be in the next show!

10. **Write a blog.** Share your going dry story or write about your hobby.

11. **Join a local club** – beekeeping, allotments, save the dolphins – there are hundreds of things out there to investigate.

12. **Go for afternoon tea.** Treat a friend or family member with some of that new extra cash.

13. **Learn a language** – use a language lab or an online course so you'll be able to say a few words in the local lingo on your next holiday abroad.

14. **Go to the cinema.** Whether it's the latest blockbuster or indy directorial debut, head out to experience something different.

15. **Visit a comedy club.** Alcohol Change UK started a trend of 'Dry Humour' comedy evenings a couple of years ago so laughing your socks off without a drink is definitely doable. You could even get a stand-up slot yourself.

16. **Visit an auction.** Whether you're bidding or not, there are some fascinating auctions taking place around the country. Whether you've got a penchant for vintage bric-a-brac or enjoy drooling over classic cars, this is a great opportunity to get up close and personal with items that you don't see on general sale. You might even nab a bargain.

17. **Parachute jump.** Believe me, if you choose this option you'll be soooo glad you haven't got a hangover when you jump.

18. **Learn something on YouTube.** There are tutorials on pretty much everything from cat midwifery to finger bopping (look it up).

19. **Write something.** Be it fiction, poetry, your memoir, a letter to a friend. Anything at all.

20. **Check out the history of your area** at your local library (if it's still open) or on the internet.

21. **Join a choir.** Even if you only ever sing in the shower, with a bit of practice you could be belting out a song like a pro. Plus, you'll meet some interesting people.

22. **Read a classic.** From Asimov to Zola, now's your chance to settle down to read some of those books you've been meaning to get round to for years.

23. **Join a gym.** Why not? If you've got more energy, you could use it getting into shape. Already a member? Why not actually go, then? Total gym lover already? You could try something different – kickboxing or Zumba, for example.

24. **Try origami.** You just need to master one complex figure to amaze your friends, charm small children and delight elderly relatives.

25. **Get your first aid certificate.** St John Ambulance runs weekend courses all over the country and the skills you learn could save a life.

26. **Listen to a podcast.** There are so many brilliant ones to choose from no matter what you're interested in. But if you really can't find the perfect one, set up your own!

27. **Learn to ride a horse.** If you can already ride – try a unicycle!

28. **Take a train trip** to somewhere new. Choose a destination at random if you're feeling spontaneous!

29. **Play a board game.** I bet when you were a kid you loved those good old-fashioned games like Cluedo, Monopoly and Scrabble. Personally I still love Kerplunk! If you can't find anyone to join you – try solitaire.

30. **Go to a pizza-making evening.** I treated my brother to a pizza-making event once and then offered him and his pizza a lift afterwards. Only one of them made it home.

31. **Do that one thing** you've always wanted to do, but haven't had the guts to. It's now or never, my friend!

By the way, if you're thinking that everyone else is permanently out having fun, celebrating every night of the week and you're just paddling along in their wake – don't. It's not true. We all need some down time so don't feel obliged to complete all or any of the list above. As I said in Chapter 1, you're supposed to be enjoying the challenge, not frantically trying to party (or parachute) your way through it sober.

Sometimes it's good to just kick off your shoes, grab your dressing gown and flop on the sofa for a day or a weekend – however long it takes until you feel recharged and ready to go again. In which case – back to Chapter 9 you go.

On the other hand, a dry month doesn't mean that your usual social life has to hit a dry spell, so do venture out if that's more your style. The main point is that this is an opportunity to enjoy, not suffer through, a month sober.

Natasha

'If there ever was an incentive to keep going, it's the waking up on a Saturday morning with a clear head, eager to face the day.'

—

11. WHAT'S NEXT?

Me: Wow. A whole month. We did it!

Myself: Of course we did. I never doubted us.

I: . . . Sure. So, what have we learned?

Me: Well, I'm surprised at how much other people drink. I'd never noticed before.

Myself: That's because they're fun and interesting.

I: Apart from when they're loud and obnoxious, you mean.

Me: And I didn't realise that we were sleeping so badly until we had our first full night of uninterrupted sleep.

Myself: True, that was heavenly.

I: The question is, what are we going to do now?

If you're almost at the end of your dry month – what's next?

If you've loved Trying Dry you might be thinking about staying dry for longer.

Or you may want to go back to drinking immediately.

Or, if you're like most past Try Dryers, you're somewhere in between – not wanting to go back to exactly how you were drinking before, but not sure you want to stay dry either.

This chapter will help you work out which camp you fall into, and how to go about it safely and happily.

Stu

'At the end of my Dry October I was pleased with my achievement and I decided that I'd try to do it again for January. I didn't make a conscious decision to go out on 1 November and get drunk, but actually I did go out, had two beers and was extremely drunk. What it made me think was, "Wow, some nights I would have eight beers and not be as drunk as I was after those two."

'The feeling of being drunk like that – it's not very nice. Now when I'm feeling like I'm kind of on the edge and the next drink is going to lead to four more, I think back to that moment on 1 November and I think, "Actually, I don't want that."'

REFLECTING ON YOUR MONTH

Do you remember that postcard that you wrote to yourself in Chapter 1? I hope you didn't write anything rude on it because it's time to take a look at the words you wanted the one-month-later you to read. How does that compare to how you're feeling now? Better? Worse? Exactly what you expected?

→ Tick the results you noticed during your Try Dry month below and see how they shape up.

	✔		✔
I've lost weight		I have more free time	
I've got more energy		I tried a new activity	
My thoughts are clearer		I gave dry dating a go	
My physical health problems improved		I tried sober sex	
I got through a tough time without a drink		I enjoyed a night out without alcohol	
My mental health problems improved		My relationship with my partner is better	
My moods have stabilised		My relationship with my children is improved	
I saved money		My relationship with friends is better	
I noticed clearer skin		I'm proud of myself	
I have fewer aches and pains		I achieved another goal, which was _____	
I'm happier at work		I've got less/no acid reflux	

I've been able to reduce my medication		I've had fewer coughs and colds	
I broke the habit of automatically reaching for a drink		I tackled a big event alcohol-free	
I have fewer/no headaches		I found an alcohol-free drink I really enjoy	
I've been complimented by friends and family		I inspired others to Try Dry	
I beat a craving		My sleep improved	
I've been doing more exercise		My hair and nails have improved	
I've got my weekends back		I've stopped procrastinating	
I'm learning to practise mindfulness		My sugar cravings have reduced	

Now compare this with your aims at the beginning of the month. Which of the following sentences best describes you:

- I got exactly what I wanted from my dry month – or maybe more!

- It wasn't as beneficial as I'd hoped.

- Help! I really couldn't manage it.

I GOT EXACTLY WHAT I WANTED – OR MAYBE MORE!

If you enjoyed the rewards and even identified benefits you hadn't considered, you're one of the thousands of Try Dry alumni who now know that a month off the booze can be a life-changing experience.

What would you like to keep from your dry month?

If you wanted this month to kick-start a healthier lifestyle, you've probably already made other changes towards your health goals. Think about where alcohol fits in with that in the future.

If you're losing weight and want to continue with that, your new dry aim might be to keep going until you have reached a healthy weight that you feel happy with (and that means not too thin too). After that, you might want to cut down going forward, and make this part of a healthier lifestyle.

On the other hand, if you just wanted to take a break to reset your drinking at a lower level, you'll be more interested in keeping track of your drinking from hereon in, so you can start to enjoy it again without some of the downsides that made you take a month off in the first place.

Download one of the drink tracker apps in the resources section in the back of the book so that you can keep an eye on what and when you're drinking. I'd obviously recommend the Dry January app, which works year-round to help you track your drinking days and units, plus money and calories saved. You'll also get articles from the Dry January team to help keep you motivated!

Mark

'Less depression is just gold for me. I don't want to use the word "life-changing" loosely but I'm shocked at the impact on my mental health.'

—

Cadence

'It gave me a breathing space. I had a chance to get to know myself on my own for the first time in my life.'

—

Grace

'Being able to go out to a pub and NOT drink alcohol has been empowering and reassuring. I no longer yearn for a pint after a busy day.'

—

IT WASN'T AS BENEFICIAL AS I HOPED

If you haven't noticed any difference, or haven't seen as many benefits as you hoped, get a second opinion. As I mentioned in Chapter 5, when Mr B Tried Dry he steadfastly refused to see any benefits until they were pointed out to him and then he realised that, actually, he was thinner, sweeter and more bouncy by the end of the month.

Ask your nearest and dearest to give you their perspective on your alcohol-free month. You are not to contradict, deny or refute any of their claims. If you're going to ask, you've got to be prepared to hear them out. After all, they have to put up with you whether you're drinking or not, so they should get a chance to have their views heard.

Not drinking for a month isn't a cure-all. Everyone is different. So while you may know people who were sleeping like a baby from day 2 and who looked ten years younger by day 20, that's not going to be everyone's experience. Rest assured, though, that your month off will have given your insides a break, even if it's not showing up on the outside.

If you completed the AUDIT quiz in Chapter 2 and scored less than 8, it's probably because booze wasn't having a big impact on your life in the first place. That doesn't mean it won't have had any benefits though; you've reset your relationship with alcohol. This will help you to drink the drinks you really enjoy and look forward to and skip the rest. That's good for your body, your brain and your wallet.

HELP! I REALLY COULDN'T MANAGE IT

Lots of people find their first attempt at a dry month is a struggle and might go through the 'reset' process several times before everything clicks into place. If this is you, flick back to Chapter 7 and see what you can do to reflect on how these setbacks went.

Was it external factors like stresses or internal cravings that made it difficult? When you work out what made staying dry so hard, you'll be better equipped to tackle it next time.

If this just wasn't the right time for you to do this challenge – that's OK. Give it a go again a few months down the line. Think about the cycle of change, though – what did you learn, good and bad, from whatever dry time you did manage? Write it down because this will be useful information for next time you go dry.

It may be that you feel you need a bit more support cutting down on your drinking. There's plenty out there and sensible people like you make use of it. Talking through your concerns and getting some strategies from a professional is a really, really good idea. If you had a blocked drain and, despite spending Sunday afternoon up to your elbows in unidentified brown sludge, it stayed stubbornly blocked, you'd call a plumber, right? Same thing.

So where is this support and what does it involve? There are a tonne of options available, and I bet there's one that would suit you.

Alcohol support services don't recommend abstinence *unless that's what you want to achieve* but they do have loads of strategies for cutting down, making changes and helping you to get where you want to go, booze-wise.

In case you're wondering, you don't necessarily have to attend appointments in person – you can now get support via Skype, apps, online courses and a whole heap of other ways that would have been unthinkable ten years ago. What have you got to lose, except the booze?

If you'd like some help, you can visit the Alcohol Change UK website, or visit your GP and ask for some advice. They can help you to consider your options and point you in the right direction.

If you're not ready to look for professional help, why not join one of the wonderful supportive online communities that offer advice and inspiration? You can find a selection in the resources section.

WHAT NEXT?

Whether you're thrilled with your new-found energy, svelte physique and bulging wallet, or still having trouble seeing the benefits, it's worth having a proper think about what's next for you and your drinking.

Here's an opportunity to jot down what alcohol gives and what it takes away. This will help you to decide how you want to proceed when your challenge is over. Can you keep some of the good things about drinking and ditch some of the bad? The perspective of a month clear of alcohol will help you to decide what longer-term changes (if any) you want to make.

→ The good things about drinking are . . .

→ The bad things about drinking are . . .

STAYING DRY

If this has been a turning point for you and you'd like to stay booze-free for the foreseeable future, you've got off to a good start! I've got just a few final tips to help keep you on track.

Keep doing what you've been doing. By now, you've probably faced going out, staying in, celebrations, weekends, down days, pay days and everything else that a month can throw at you. Take some time to think about the tough and tempting times and how you overcame them. And stay focused. It's easy to revert to habit when your mind is elsewhere.

Don't think about for ever – think a day, a week or a month at a time. Breaking it down into smaller chunks is always less daunting. You don't even need to set a goal – just take each day as it comes and decide as you go along. I've not considered the idea of 'never' drinking again. I just don't drink. I'm free to change that decision any time I want and that takes the pressure off.

Why not join an online sober community such as Dry January and Beyond on Facebook, Club Soda or Soberistas? They're full of inspirational people, just like you, who no longer drink. You'll pick up tips and ideas and share stories of dry life to keep you motivated over the coming weeks. If all else fails, at least you'll have a whole new group of people to admire photos of your grandchild/cat/new skateboard.

Go back to Chapter 1 to remind yourself of why you want to stay off the booze for a bit longer. Chapters 9 and 10 will also help you with drink ideas and ways to continue to have fun without a drink in your hand.

→ Write why you want to continue to stay dry here:

GOING DAMP

You'd like to drink again but not at the levels you were drinking before your dry month. If you'd like to set the bar (geddit?) a little lower, it will help to keep a diary of your drinking days so you can see if the amount you're drinking starts to creep up. There are several free apps that will help you to do this, including the Dry January app, OneYou Drink Tracker and DrinkCoach.

You can use an app or try the calculation in Chapter 2 to work out how many units you were drinking before you started your challenge and decide how many you'd like to be drinking from now on. Spend a few minutes working out how many drinks this means and plan each week's drinking to keep you at your chosen level.

→ Write how often and how much you'll be drinking from now on here:

Lily

'My drinking is absolutely lower than it was before. In fact, I know it's never going to be the same. The thing that was so great about the end of Dry January was that I wanted to keep going. That was powerful.'

→ Cutting down is quite a different skill to cutting out, and it's worth thinking about some methods you can use to do so. In the table below, jot down some ways that you might be able to reduce your drinking. Put down at least ten. Really.

Now decide how easy or hard it would be to put your strategy into practice and why and give each one a score out of ten, with ten being extremely difficult and one being a piece of cake (sorry, can't help myself).

Choose a strategy with a low score, say four or lower, and try it out for a couple of weeks. If it's going well, pick another strategy to add on top. If it bombed, choose another option to try. Move your way up through the strategies towards the ones with a higher score until you're happy you've made enough changes.

Ways I can cut down my drinking	How easy/difficult will this be?	Score
e.g. I could avoid going to the pub.	Hard. I work there three nights a week.	9

My top tip for going damp is to think about what drinks you really enjoy and look forward to, and only drink those. Maybe you're really only a white wine guy, but often find yourself drinking other things because they're there. Ditch the rest and drink only the things you love.

This tip works well for special occasions too; it's Christmas Day and you LOVE having a mulled wine in the evening, but you can do without the Buck's Fizz in the morning, wine at lunch and Auntie Sally's famous elderberry gin all afternoon. Well – savour the mulled wine, skip the rest, and enjoy your clear head the next day!

WET AT WEEKENDS

If you'd noticed your drinking creeping up to almost every day and you'd like to save it as a special treat for weekends and special occasions, this is the way forward. Lots of people find this a comfortable way of maintaining lower levels of drinking without feeling that they have to go without. Setting rules, such as only drinking on Fridays and Saturdays, makes your plan easier to stick to. As long as you can avoid adding in caveats and exceptions, you should find it straightforward.

Just because you're only drinking at weekends doesn't mean you should go crazy on Friday and Saturday; the UK's low-risk drinking guidelines recommend a maximum of 14 units a week, spread over several days (i.e. not 14 units all on one night).

Make a note of your plans for weekends here.

➜ I'll make sure I only drink at weekends by . . .

Andrew

'The Six Nations before would be "watch the rugby with friends, get a bit tipsy on a Saturday afternoon". This year watching it, for the first time ever, I had a load of Nanny State alcohol-free beer in the fridge. And I drank that while watching Saturday-afternoon rugby. If you'd told me 12 months ago I'd be doing that I'd have laughed you out of the room.

'I've got a much different take on things. I have returned to enjoying an alcoholic drink rather than needing an alcoholic drink. There are certain occasions where I would habitually have an alcoholic drink and it works equally well for me now to not have a beer in my hand. I would never, never have thought that would be me.'

DIVING STRAIGHT BACK IN

Dry month done and you're all set to get back to normal. Stop right there!

After a month of not drinking, your body and brain have got used to no booze and your tolerance for the stuff has diminished. So you need to start drinking again slowly. You'll find that it takes much less booze to get you 'mellow' so plan accordingly. Drinking the way you used to, getting totally wasted and feeling rubbish for the next two days . . . I'd respectfully suggest that's a bad idea.

Try deciding in advance how much you'd like to be drinking and working your way up to it rather than getting straight back to your old drinking level. Another tip: it's OK to refuse a drink now and then. Don't just drink because it's there: positively choose it and enjoy it!

To make sure that you don't go overboard at first, plan to drink a soft drink between every alcoholic drink for a couple of weeks: it'll slow you down and help with the hangover.

On the rare occasions when I've dabbled with drinking, I've made sure it's just one drink, and that's plenty. I recall a particular spa break in Spain when I thought I'd get my money's worth and order the free hotel bar cocktail that came as part of the package. I don't know what was in it but I suspect it was five parts tequila to one part lemonade. Three sips later and I'm singing 'Una Paloma Blanca' at the top of my voice. Luckily, the astute Mr B had shepherded me back to the room by then; just in time for me to tell him how much I bloody love him and pass out on the patio. He has photos. That's why I can never leave him.

If you drink at home, it can be hard to work out how much you drink. What you call a 'glass' might be described as a bucket by someone else, so here's a handy tip: pour your usual amount into your regular glass, then tip the glass into a measuring jug. Use the calculation in Chapter 2 to discover how many units are in your usual tipple. I did this activity with someone recently and we found out that his usual 'one drink' was actually *seven* units! If this sounds like you, I definitely recommend getting smaller glasses.

If you generally drink when out at pubs and clubs, one of the apps at the back of the book will help you to work out how many units are in a pub measure of your chosen drink.

TIPS FROM THE TOP

Whatever you decide to do now that your month is over, here are some great tips from other Try Dryers to help keep you on track.

- 'Download an app to keep track of your units and how many calories you're drinking, it helps you stick to just the drinks you really want.'

- 'Write down what you liked about your dry month and put it somewhere you can see it every day, to remind yourself of your achievement.'

- 'Go forward with a friend. Find someone with the same goal as you and support each other.'

- 'Join an online community.'

- 'Keep a journal.'

- 'Plan in another dry month.'

- 'Read some of the inspirational books by people who've gained control of their drinking or given up completely.'

- 'Set yourself a longer dry challenge. Three months? A year?'

SO LONG FOR NOW

Well, that's it. We've come to the end of our dry adventure together.

Don't worry, I'm not leaving you high and dry (ahem). There are so many people, organisations, forums, apps and communities that can help as you go forward.

Whether you're a total convert and planning to be dry for ever, or want to get back to how you were before, I reckon your dry month will have made a difference to how you think and feel about alcohol.

If you've been inspired, ignited or just plain blown away by your Try Dry challenge, don't keep it to yourself. Pass this book on, inspire others, write a blog, open a dry bar, brew a brilliant booze-free beer. You've already done one amazing thing this month; don't stop there.

If you're reading ahead and haven't actually done your month – what are you waiting for? This is it, the end of the book, nothing more to see here, so no more procrastinating – go and Try Dry!

MY TRY DRY CHALLENGE PLAN

My reasons for taking a dry month are (see page 21):

1. _____

_____

2. _____

_____

3. _____

_____

My challenge begins on (date) _____ (see page 37)

It will finish on (date) _____

I will save £_____ over the next month (see page 41)

I'm going to spend all that lovely money on _____

My alcohol-free drink of the month is _____
(see page 168)

These people will be my supporters (see page 54)

_____

_____

_____

_____

These are my sober buddies (see page 57)

_____

_____

_____

_____

My elevator pitch is (see page 52)

_____

_____

_____

_____

_____

_____

_____

THOUGHT FOR THE DAY

Past Try Dryers have said that a little something every day really helps to keep the momentum up. So here are 31 'thoughts for the day' to see you through.

1. Welcome to your challenge. In just four weeks you will have joined the growing community who have taken a month off booze. Enjoy the ride!

2. Have you thought about what you're going to drink tonight? If you normally have a welcome home drink, a glass of something with dinner or a small nightcap to help you drop off, then it's worth thinking up some delicious alcohol-free alternatives. Herbal tea, anyone?

3. Better sleep, more energy, healthier hair and skin, weight loss and a bit more money in your pocket are just some of the benefits that people report after a month off booze. Plus you'll be doing a lot of good for your insides too. That's not a bad way to spend a month.

4. How are you getting on? You'll be pleased to hear that after just three days, your body is already feeling the difference and all the grog is likely to be out of your system by now.

5. If you haven't already, why not download the Dry January app for some extra tips along the way? Check out the full list of helpful apps in the resources section.

6. Are you drinking lots of water? It's easy to rely on alcohol to quench your thirst so why not treat yourself to a sports water bottle and make sure you get your two litres a day.

7. Plan something fun for this evening so that you're not at a loose end and have something to look forward to.

8. You've done a whole week! Remember to complete your first weekly check-in.

9. Give yourself a big pat on the back and a little treat – you're over a quarter of the way through your challenge.

10. How are you sleeping? If you've been struggling to nod off without a drink, take heart – your natural sleep pattern should be kicking in around now!

11. You should be in the swing of things by now and feeling the benefits of ten days alcohol-free. Have you become the 'Wow, I feel amazing' office bore yet? Good for you. Ignore them, they're just jealous.

12. If you found your first booze-free weekend a bit of a challenge, you'll be delighted to hear that the second one should be easier. After all, you know you can do it now.

13. There are few things as motivating as hearing inspirational stories from other people on the same journey. Why not flick through the book and read how some other Try Dryers tackled their dry month?

14. Wow, two weeks. Well done, you. I hope you're feeling amazing – but if you're not, that's OK too. It can take your body a while to adjust. Stick with it!

15. Is it that time already? Two weeks in so time to think about completing your weekly check-in again.

16. How are you feeling? By now, the extra energy and better sleep might be starting to kick in. But if not, stay with it. If you're wavering at all, look back at your original motivations.

17. OK, I've done all the work so far – it's time you contributed. Make up your own bloody thought for the day.

18. What's the weirdest thing you've noticed during your two and a half weeks without a drink? Any unexpected benefits? Answers on a postcard please.

19. Have you looked at your Try Dry challenge plan lately? Why not take a quick peek to remind yourself what you wrote down to help you on your journey.

20. Part of breaking old habits is replacing them with new ones. Now is the perfect time to embark on a new adventure.

21. Day 21 already. Three whole weeks – that's quite an achievement. How are you going to celebrate? Time to introduce a new treat!

22. Between more energy, fewer nights having the same pub-fuelled conversation and no mornings lost to hangovers, you're probably feeling pretty incredible by now and you're two-thirds of the way through the month. If you're struggling, now's the time to push yourself. You can do it!

23. Congratulations. It can take as little as three weeks to break a habit and by now you should be finding the going easier and the benefits more apparent.

24. What if you haven't noticed any benefits yet? Why not ask your friends and family what they've noticed about you since you started your challenge?

25. Why not contact an old friend that you haven't been in touch with for a while and arrange to go for a coffee?

26. Three and a half weeks. I'm soooo proud! Has anyone asked you how you've done it, yet? Why not lend them the book so they can give it a try too?

27. As we head towards the end of the month, it's time to start thinking about what happens next. FYI, 72 per cent of Try Dryers have lower AUDIT scores six months later and 8 per cent don't go back to the booze at all.

28. So, here we are, nearly at the end. How's it been? Easier than you expected? Harder? Time to complete your weekly check-in again.

29. How are you feeling? By now you should have some idea whether you want to continue to stay off the booze or ease yourself back in. Either way, rest assured that your body is delighted that you've taken a dry month.

30. Remember that postcard you wrote to yourself back at the beginning of the month? Well now is the time to take a look at what old you wanted to say to new you.

31. Have you danced sober yet? If not, why not give it a try tonight. If today is a midweek day, there's still no excuse not to turn up the radio and jump around your living room, just for the hell of it. After all, you're celebrating the final day of your challenge. Big pat on the back from us and sparkling water all round. Cheers!

RESOURCES

BLOGS

The Dry Blog

www.alcoholchange.org.uk

Dry January's very own blog, with hot tips, inspiring stories and more. You can sign up to Dry January from this page, too.

Girl & Tonic

www.girlandtonic.co.uk

Laurie McAllister is a 20-something blogging about her life in Norfolk, yoga and not drinking. Some great articles (including what to do after your Try Dry challenge) and a bit of yoga thrown in for good measure.

Living Sober

www.livingsober.org.nz

Funny, heartfelt posts from blogger Mrs D and her community. 'I used to be a boozy housewife. Now I'm not.' This is the only non-British blog on the list. Not that there aren't many wonderful inspirational international resources, but space is limited so go and find your own world blogs.

Mummy Was a Secret Drinker

mummywasasecretdrinker.blogspot.com

Author of *The Sober Diaries*, Clare Pooley's blog was where it all started for her. After a year of anonymous blogging, Clare has stepped out of the closet and shares fantastic advice on your Try Dry journey. Check out her TEDx Talk, too.

Undrunk

grahamwilsonundrunk.com

Graham Wilson has been blogging since 2016 about mental health, recovery and men's health. He wants everyone, men especially, to know that 'It's OK to say you're not OK.'

ONLINE COMMUNITIES

Club Soda

www.clubsoda.co.uk

A mindful drinking movement with lots of resources, courses and events, including festivals, workshops and monthly alcohol-free lunches in cities around the country. The website posts events where booze isn't front and centre and the monthly socials are great for meeting others who are also giving dry a try.

One Year No Beer

www.oneyearnobeer.com

Fellas, you'll love this one. OYNB is run by two former hard-drinking chaps who've embraced a sober lifestyle and offer challenges from 28 days to the full one year without beer (or wine, or whatever). Great podcasts, too.

Soberistas

www.soberistas.com

An online community of alcohol-free members offering information, support, personal stories and lots of humour, warmth and acceptance. This is the website for you if you're looking for some sober support throughout your challenge.

Dry January Facebook group

This is our very own closed Facebook group for anyone who's done, doing or thinking about taking a Dry January. It's a friendly, supportive community of like-minded people sharing woes and successes.

PLACES TO BUY NON-ALCOHOLIC DRINKS

Dry Drinker

www.drydrinker.com

Craft beers, sparkling wines and even pink gin. This fantastic website has over 100 alcohol-free beers, wines and spirits to deliver right to your door the very next day. Nice.

The Alcohol-Free Shop

www.alcoholfree.co.uk

Order online from these veterans of the alcohol-free scene, who have been selling non-alcoholic drinks for over ten years. They claim to have 'served everyone from rock stars, to 'residents of Number 10', actors and footballers'.

APPS

DrinkCoach

A lovely app that has a mindfulness video and a craving diary.

Dry January

Not just for January. You can use this all year round to track units, drink-free days, money and calories saved and more, plus access great articles from the Dry January team.

Leaf

Leaf lets you track your drinks and offers a monthly challenge whether you're cutting down or cutting out the booze.

OneYou Drinks Tracker

Part of the OneYou series from the NHS, this is a unit tracker that gives you the unit guidelines and tips and advice for making changes to your drinking. There are Couch to 5K, healthy eating and Smoke free OneYou apps too. Why not collect the set?

Headspace

A great mindfulness app with guided meditations on different themes, depending on what you need at the time, that take just a few minutes each day.

Insight Timer

Another great mindfulness app with different topics and even podcasts. One great feature is that you can see how many people are doing the exercise with you. Very Zen, dudes.

FURTHER READING

The Unexpected Joy of Being Sober

Catherine Gray

Catherine's candid story of her drinking problem and her sobriety. The second half of the book contains fantastic tips on everything from sober sex to dealing with heartbreak. This is a great read.

The 28 Day Alcohol-Free Challenge

Andy Ramage and Ruari Fairbairns

From the amazing guys at One Year No Beer. This is a brilliant one-month alcohol-free challenge book and companion to the website.

The Sober Diaries

Clare Pooley

Funny, heartwarming and real. Clare's story (yes, Clare of blog Mummy Was a Secret Drinker) will resonate with every parent who's ever had to juggle a toddler and a hangover at the same time. Not literally, of course.

This Naked Mind

Annie Grace

This book explains why we're all so hung up on drink. Many, many people have given up the booze, at least for a while, after reading this book.

At Alcohol Change UK, they're always looking for great ideas to spice up the list of resources (they're also a big help to the annual Dry January campaign) – so if there's anything you want to share, whether it's blogs, wisdom, anecdotes, dry ideas, sober stories or you just plain want to chat, why not get in touch?

SPECIAL THANKS

First of all, I'd like to thank my husband, Andrew, for the love (and the cake).

Next, the whole team at Alcohol Change UK, for their work to help us all to drink more happily and healthily. As it stands, alcohol does so much more harm than good in the UK, and Alcohol Change UK are working to end that harm. They do that through Dry January, but so much more besides. You can find out more about them on their website.

Heartfelt thanks go to Maddy Lawson at Alcohol Change UK for believing in this book. You never doubted that it could be done and did all the organising, liaising, negotiating, chivvying and editing that made the idea a reality. You are a star.

A massive thank you to all the Try Dryers who lent their stories to this book to help others starting out on their own dry journeys. You're brave, brilliant and so appreciated.

Thank you to Lee Mack, for contributing your witty, thought-provoking foreword, your insight into the world of television alcohol advertising, and for your ongoing support of Alcohol Change UK.

To Dr Chris Record, thank you for using your expertise to review the medical information in Chapter 5.

The team at Square Peg have been amazing. Harriet Dobson and Rowan Yapp have guided us through the slightly terrifying process of writing a book with patience and sensitivity – thank you.

There are so many more people to thank, because Dry January (and so *Try Dry*) brings in so many people to make it the campaign it is. To everyone who has organised an event for Dry January in your community or workplace, put up posters to tell people about it, shared it on social media . . . thank you.

And finally thank YOU, for buying this book. You're helping to fund Alcohol Change UK's lifesaving work – plus you're part of a HUGE and growing movement of people taking control of their relationship with alcohol by Trying Dry. High five.

ALCOHOL CHANGE UK

Try Dry and Dry January are brought to you by the charity **Alcohol Change UK**. We work for a society that is free from the harm caused by alcohol.

Alcohol is a part of many of our lives. We use it for celebration, for comfort, to socialise, to wind down, to cope. It's legal, socially acceptable, even encouraged. Yet in the UK one person every hour dies as a result of alcohol. Alcohol harm – mental health problems, liver disease, six forms of cancer, economic difficulties, and so much more – can affect any one of us, from any walk of life. And each of us who drinks too much is part of a family and a community who feel the effects too.

We are not anti-alcohol; we are for alcohol change. We are for a future in which people drink as a conscious choice, not a default; where the issues which lead to alcohol problems – like poverty, mental health problems, homelessness – are addressed; where those of us who drink too much, and our loved ones, have access to high-quality support whenever we need it, without shame or stigma.

The problem is complex, so the solutions aren't simple. But we're ambitious. Driven by our belief that every person deserves to live free from alcohol harm, we create smart, evidence-driven change.

Find out more about alcohol harm or join us to make change happen faster at **alcoholchange.org.uk**

MY TRY DRY NOTES